D1385223

PRAISE FOR

What to Eat When You Want to Get Pregnant

"Science shows that nutrition impacts not only the ability to conceive, but also contributes greatly to a healthy pregnancy. Neuroscientist Dr. Nicole Avena gives both women and men the information they need to optimize their fertility as well as their own long-term health. Anyone who is trying to have a baby, is thinking about it, or dealing with fertility issues needs to read this book."
—**Sara Gottfried, MD,** *New York Times* bestselling author
 of *The Hormone Cure*

"A comprehensive guide to nutrition and reproduction. The necessary follow-up to her vital book, *What to Eat When You're Pregnant,* this current work elevates the importance of nutrition to not only improve fertility but also the pregnancy journey and its outcome . . . Dr. Avena successfully takes on the daunting task of simplifying the current scientific data to empower the reader. I will add this book to my recommendations of important resources for my patients."
—**Mark P. Trolice, MD, FACOG, FACS, FACE,**
 director, Fertility CARE: The IVF Center

"Where was this book when I was trying to get pregnant? Lucky for you, it is now available thanks to Dr. Nicole Avena, an expert I admire in health and neuroscience. *What to Eat When You Want to Get Pregnant* will give you science-based solutions to boost your fertility and health leading up to and during parenthood."
—**Laurie David,** author, environmental advocate,
 producer of *An Inconvenient Truth*

"*What to Eat When You Want to Get Pregnant* is exactly the book I want to share with my patients who are contemplating pregnancy or facing infertility. In a conversational, easy-to-follow style, Dr. Nicole Avena provides her readers with a well-researched, easy-to-follow, and comprehensive approach to optimizing the diet and eating habits of hopeful moms as well as dads. With a strong background in both nutrition and psychology, Dr. Avena is an ideal guide for those seeking to boost their chances of a healthy pregnancy."
—**Sarah Samaan, MD, FACC**

"Science shows that nutrition impacts not only the ability to conceive, but also contributes to a healthy pregnancy. Dr. Nicole Avena gives both women and men the information they need to optimize their fertility as well as their own long-term health. Everyone who wants to have a baby at some point—and particularly women who are actively trying to have one right now—need to read this book."
—**Katherine Ryder,** founder and CEO of Maven

"As a nutrition expert and mom, this book will be on my must-read list for every woman I know looking to optimize their diet for fertility."
—**Patricia Bannan, MS, RDN,** nationally recognized nutritionist
  and healthy-cooking expert

"Practical strategies and healthy eating guides for men and women who will now have a marvelous and valuable tool to use nutrition to boost fertility."
—**Dr. Michael Goren,** professor of pediatrics
  at Children's Hospital, Los Angeles

"Given the increasing challenges to achieving (and maintaining) a healthy pregnancy, Nicole Avena's immensely useful and readable *What to Eat When You Want to Get Pregnant* is just the book we need right now . . . Full of humor, practical advice on foods to eat (and avoid), and recipes to prepare them, every young couple trying to conceive will want to buy (and frequently refer to) this valuable resource."
—**Dr. Shanna Swan,** author of *Count Down: How Our Modern World
  Is Threatening Sperm Counts, Altering Male and Female Reproductive Health,
  and Imperiling the Future of the Human Race*

"There's nothing more heartbreaking than wanting a baby but not being able to conceive. While we do have assisted reproductive technologies, what about do-it-yourself? Way more effective, and way more fun. Dr. Avena has assembled the science of nutrition and fertility in one place to help your chances for success."
—**Robert H. Lustig, MD, MSL,** University of California, San Francisco

"You can't always control how quickly you will get pregnant, but you can improve your chances of a healthy pregnancy through lifestyle choices and nutrition. Dr. Avena's latest book, which walks through the Four-Week Fertility-Boosting Plan, is well-researched and easy to follow. I highly recommend this book for people in the TTC (trying to conceive) journey to better understand how fertility and nutrition are intertwined, and what you can do to optimize your chances."
—**Halle Tecco,** CEO, Natalist

"*What to Eat When You Want to Get Pregnant* offers an evidence-based and user-friendly program to boost fertility. If you want to have a baby, read this book!"
—**Lisa Young, PhD, RDN,** author of *Finally Full, Finally Slim*
  and adjunct professor of nutrition at NYU

"I love this book! Dr. Nicole Avena provides a wealth of trustworthy guidance about fertility-boosting nutrition in a friendly and easy-to-access format. This book also incorporates important tips on ways to avoid unwelcome toxic chemicals that lurk in the kitchen and can be harmful to a woman's health and pregnancy. A wonderful resource for moms-to-be!"
—**Alexandra Destler, EdM,** founder and CEO, SafetyNEST

"This is the only book of its kind, because alongside the hard science, Dr. Avena also provides practical advice gleaned from her experience as a mother of two children."
—**Dr. Vera Tarman,** author of *Food Junkies: Recovery from Food Addiction*

What to Eat When You Want to Get Pregnant

A Science-Based Four-Week Program
to Boost Your Fertility with Nutrition

● ● ● ● ● ● ● ● ● ● ● ● ● ●

Nicole M. Avena, PhD

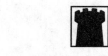

CITADEL PRESS
Kensington Publishing Corp.
www.kensingtonbooks.com

CITADEL PRESS BOOKS are published by

Kensington Publishing Corp.
119 West 40th Street
New York, NY 10018

Copyright © 2021 Nicole M. Avena

All rights reserved. No part of this book may be reproduced in any form or by any means without the prior written consent of the publisher, excepting brief quotes used in reviews.

PUBLISHER'S NOTE
This book is sold to readers with the understanding that while the publisher aims to inform, enlighten, and provide accurate general information regarding the subject matter covered, the publisher is not engaged in providing medical, psychological, financial, legal, or other professional services. If the reader needs or wants professional advice or assistance, the services of an appropriate professional should be sought. Case studies featured in this book are composites based on the author's years of practice and do not reflect the experiences of any individual person.

All Kensington titles, imprints, and distributed lines are available at special quantity discounts for bulk purchases for sales promotions, premiums, fund-raising, educational, or institutional use.

Special book excerpts or customized printings can also be created to fit specific needs. For details, write or phone the office of the Kensington sales manager: Kensington Publishing Corp., 119 West 40th Street, New York, NY 10018, attn: Sales Department; phone 1-800-221-2647.

CITADEL PRESS and the Citadel logo are Reg. U.S. Pat. & TM Off.

ISBN-13: 978-0-8065-4070-2
ISBN-10: 0-8065-4070-2

First Citadel hardcover printing: April 2021

10 9 8 7 6 5 4 3 2 1

Printed in the United States of America

Library of Congress Control Number: 2020945346

Electronic edition:

ISBN-13: 978-0-8065-4072-6 (e-book)
ISBN-10: 0-8065-4072-9 (e-book)

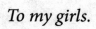

To my girls.

Contents

PART I

What You Need to Know About Nutrition and Getting Pregnant Today

CHAPTER 1

So You Want to Have a Baby . . .

Congratulations! If you have picked up this book, you are likely getting ready to embark on the magical journey of parenthood. Maybe you are just in the beginning stages of thinking about "trying," or maybe you have been trying for a while and are willing to do anything at this point to get pregnant, and are turning to this book for some additional help to get you there. Either way, I can relate: I have been in both places.

Before I get into my story, let me back up a little and tell you a little bit about myself. I am a neuroscientist and work in the fields of addiction and nutrition. I have a special interest in understanding how the things we ingest, like drugs or foods, affect the brain (including the developing brain), and my lab has been doing research on this topic for over fifteen years. I also have a PhD in psychology and use psychological principles to better understand why we eat certain foods and how we can change eating habits for the better.

Okay, back to my story. When my husband and I had been married for about five years, we (well, I, at first) started thinking about having a baby. I was finishing up my postdoctoral training, he was set in his career, we had put down roots in a nice town, and we had even successfully test-drove this whole "parenting" idea with a puppy. All seemed in place to add a baby into the mix. Then about two months later, I was pregnant. Piece of cake!

Then when our daughter was two years old, we started thinking it might be the right time to have another baby. This time, though, it wasn't so easy. Months of unsuccessful trying led to over a year with no luck, which ultimately led us to a reproductive endocrinologist. While we were thankful for the one beautiful baby that we had, it was still a hard time as we began on the arduous journey of treatment for secondary infertility.

There are many reasons for infertility, and in some cases, the cause is clear and there really isn't much you can do lifestyle-wise to "fix" it. However, often it isn't always clear why a couple is experiencing infertility. Since I study the effects of nutrition on health for a living, I had a pretty healthy lifestyle to begin with, but when I wasn't able to get pregnant, and the doctors didn't have a good answer as to why this was happening, I started asking myself if there was something that I could do, or not do, to make things happen? I started paying even more careful attention to the research studies that were out there about fertility. And I started to take a very critical look at what I was eating and putting in (and on) my body, and realized that *a lot* of it had ingredients that were potentially harmful to not only my health, but also to a growing baby. So, I started to clean up my (and my husband's) diet and lifestyle even more. And, eventually, we had our second daughter.

I wanted to write this book because I want to share what I learned and know, both as a scientist who studies nutrition and as a woman who has gone through the struggles, frustrations, setbacks, and ultimate joy that can sometimes come when you want to get pregnant. Of all of the things I learned, one thing stands out: While often feeling like I had *no control* over what was happening, I learned that *you can control a lot more than you think*, and your hormones and health are *not* completely out of your control. The scary part was that many of the everyday things, like what we eat ("we" meaning you *and* your partner) can have a significant impact on our health *and* our ability to have a baby.

There are tons of new research studies (which I will get into in later chapters) linking ingredients in certain foods to infertility. For example, did you know that seemingly harmless food additives like artificial sweeteners can decrease oocyte (a fancy term for an immature egg cell) quality in women, and preclinical studies suggest monosodium glutamate (MSG) may negatively impact sperm counts in men? Artificial sweeteners are everywhere—in diet sodas, flavored waters, and low-calorie or low-sugar foods, and we put them into our tea and coffee when we are trying to be "healthy" and avoid sugar. You are probably familiar with MSG, the flavor enhancer that is typically found in Chinese food, but is also often found in processed meats and some canned veggies and soups. It gives food a savory, salty flavor, often referred to as "umami." Although both are generally recognized as safe by the U.S. Food and Drug Administration (FDA), there is an abundance of research to show that perhaps this is not necessarily the case if you are trying to get pregnant.

And it isn't just food additives that we need to be concerned about. Even some foods that are considered healthy can be detrimental to fertility or pregnancy. For example, everyone loves the superfood flax, right? While it has powerful antioxidant properties and other health benefits, flaxseed oil can alter progesterone/estrogen ratios, which can be bad for trying to make a baby.

Also, it isn't just the things we eat, but also the things that come *in contact with* our food, like plastic bags and the packaging around food products, that can impact fertility. One chemical in particular, known as Surfynol, which is found in plastic, has recently been named a "reprotoxic" chemical for its ability to interfere with fertility, especially in men. But more on this, and where to look so you know how to avoid it, later.

So you are probably wondering, if all of these things are bad for us and for a baby, why the heck are they allowed to be in our food supply? The answer is complicated. When the science is mixed, or when there aren't a lot of studies out there to suggest something in *not safe*, we often assume something *is safe*. I know that sounds ridiculous, but that is how it works. The concept of being innocent until proven guilty applies to food chemicals, additives, and ingredients, just like it does to suspected criminals! Sometimes these questionable ingredients are cheap and save companies money, so companies opt to use them for economic reasons. Other times, the definite pros, like enhanced taste, texture, or food safety (i.e., some additives are used to prevent food spoilage) are believed to outweigh the potential cons. It's a complicated political battle that involves stakeholders from the food industry and the government, and it is frustrating for health experts and consumers alike.

But it isn't all bad news. There are also many studies that show that certain foods can *promote* fertility in both men and women. In later chapters, I will walk you through which foods to avoid and which to eat more of to help boost your fertility.

Making a Baby 101

You might be wondering, why do I have to worry about what I eat to get pregnant? It's just sperm + egg = baby, right? While in theory this is true, science tells us that there is a little more to it, and what you and your partner eat *can*, in fact, have an impact on how easy (or hard) it is for you to get pregnant.

Although for some it happens with ease, biologically getting pregnant is not so simple. Let's take a quick look at some stats, and review what they taught us in middle-school health class. Women typically ovulate once per cycle, which is usually around once each month. This means that one time each month, an egg is released from an ovary and travels down the fallopian tube, where we can usually expect fertilization to occur. For most women, in any given month there is a 25 percent of getting pregnant if you are having unprotected sex. But note that this percentage decreases with age, and by age 35, the odds fall close to 15–20 percent in any given month. And that is when everything is running smoothly and there aren't any known health complications or conditions impacting your fertility.

Infertility is defined as not being able to get pregnant or stay pregnant after one year of trying, or six months if you are age 35 or older. According to the Centers for Disease Control and Prevention (CDC), about 10 percent of women of child-bearing age in the United States experience infertility—that's a whopping 6.1 million women. To add insult to injury, the fertility rate among those 35–39 years old is half that of women in their 20s and early 30s, whereas the fertility rate among women above 40 is significantly reduced even further.

Despite these numbers, it's interesting to know birth rates among women age 34 and younger are decreasing, while birth rates are increasing in women over 35. This suggests that more and more women are delaying childbirth to later in life. Why? There are a variety of factors that contribute to these trends. For example, these days, women are not only pursuing careers outside of the traditional role as homemaker, many may also be settling down with a partner later in life. With this delay, however, comes a smaller window of time for a pregnancy to happen, and getting pregnant can be much, much harder.

Today, about one-third of couples with a woman over the age of 35 have fertility problems, so for these women it is important to be proactive to ensure that the first (and possibly only) attempt to have a child will be successful. However, even younger women who might not be concerned about age-related declining fertility also need to pay attention to what they are consuming before pregnancy. There is *a lot* of new research that suggests that what you eat before and during pregnancy (especially in very early pregnancy) can have a long-term impact on the health of a baby. Remember, toxins and other health-disrupting chemicals that we are often exposed to via food don't just disappear overnight. It can take months (or years in some cases) for our bodies to metabolize and excrete them.

So what should you take from all of this? To put it simply, no matter what your age or how far away you think you are from wanting to get pregnant, you need to start making lifestyle changes now, *before* becoming pregnant. The good news is that many of these changes can be easily implemented. Later in the book, I will discuss in detail why being a healthy weight, eating right, and minimizing stress and exposure to fertility-disrupting toxins, among other things, can be the secret to your success when trying to get pregnant.

Why Food Matters

To start off, let's consider one of the most basic examples of nutrition and fertility: When women don't consume enough calories on a daily basis, they eventually stop menstruating, and when women aren't menstruating, the ovaries aren't releasing eggs. Your body can flip the switch from fertile to infertile just like that. This is because our bodies know, based on our diets, when to prepare (or not) for the possibility of getting pregnant. Think about it—if you are in a famine and there is little or no food available, is it really a good time to try to get pregnant? Probably not, since if you can't support your own nutritional needs, how would you be able to support all of the extra needs that come along with carrying a baby? When our bodies sense that there is lack of food, or even certain nutrients, it is nature's way of saying that the environment is not ideal for a baby to thrive, so fertility will naturally decrease.

On the other side of the spectrum, decreased pregnancy rates are seen in women who are overweight or obese (which is defined by having a body mass index [BMI] over 25 kg/m^2). These women are also susceptible to having a higher chance of miscarriage, longer time to conception, and increased risk of pregnancy issues like premature labor, hypertension, and gestational diabetes. You might be wondering why if someone is overweight, and presumably not "starving," this would happen. The reason is simple: Being overweight or obese does not mean that one isn't starving. In fact, many individuals who struggle with obesity are also malnourished. This is because the quality of the food, not the quantity (i.e. calories), is what matters in terms of nutrition. Our bodies pick up on this just like they would if someone was underweight, and fertility will naturally decrease. Don't worry, I'll explain more about how this works in chapter 2.

While we don't often hear about it in the mainstream media, there is an overwhelming amount of research on the subject of nutrition and fertility. While there may not be a one-size-fits-all plan, the evidence-based recommendations are clear when you look at the research. For example, higher intakes of omega-3 fatty acids, folate, and fiber are consistently linked to an increased chance of getting pregnant, having a successful pregnancy, and a lower chance of suffering from infertility. For men, clinical research shows that they can add foods rich in zinc (like oysters), selenium (like sunflower seeds and certain mushrooms), and vitamin C to help improve sperm motility and mobility. These are just a few of the many examples of research on this topic, more of which will be covered throughout the book.

Just like there are recommendations, there are also warnings about foods—and particular ingredients—to avoid if you want to get pregnant. The problem is that much of this information is not widely publicized, and unless you scour the research journals, you aren't likely to hear about it. That is where I come in, to sift through the science and give you the breakdown of what the latest studies say about diet and fertility. For example, did you know that consuming too much processed meat (and red meat, too, for that matter) is a big no-no when it comes to trying to boost your fertility? Although meat can be a good source of protein and some essential vitamins and minerals such as vitamin B_{12} and iron, red and processed meats contribute to inflammation throughout the body. Inflammation plays a large role in disease, and research shows that inflammation has a negative effect on fertility and can lead to pregnancy complications.

Why This Book

We know that the prenatal environment is so important to the health and well-being of a growing baby, and there's more and more research to support the relationship between nutrition and fertility. It is never too early to start making changes in the way you eat and your mindset around food to improve your health and how you feel. Getting your body and mind in top baby-making shape can take time and isn't something that can happen overnight.

This book is filled with the latest, science-based information that is hard to find anywhere else. Everything you want to know about fertility and nutrition is covered, from specific nutrients and meal plans to how to change your eating habits (and stick to these new changes), as well as how nutrition affects male fertility and IVF success.

Not only will you walk away from this book with a plethora of knowledge related to nutrition and fertility, but you'll also have my Four-Week Fertility-Boosting Plan that you can use to guide you. The plan includes tips on what foods you should eat and avoid, in addition to ways you can easily get them in your diet via meal ideas and some fun recipes.

The Four-Week Fertility-Boosting Plan isn't just a menu, either, but a plan to help you stick to the dietary changes I recommend (which can be especially hard for some if they have been eating an unhealthy diet). The plan will help you use psychology to reduce cravings, think differently about food, and minimize stress without using food as a crutch or a way to self-medicate.

How to Use This Book

As you can see, it's becoming increasingly important to be concerned with fertility, regardless of age (or sex). Throughout this book, I will discuss everything you'll need to know about eating well for fertility, including how to successfully change your eating habits and make the right choices when grocery shopping, meal prepping, eating out, and in social situations. You'll get to know all the key nutrients associated with health and improved fertility, as well as their food sources, and the foods that you should limit (or completely avoid). Everything I am going to tell you is rooted in science; no personal-experience-that-worked-for-me-so-it-will-for-you claims here. I'll talk about research studies throughout the book, and if you are a science geek like me and want more details, you can flip to the References (page 177), where I list all of the studies and sources I refer to.

Chapter 2 starts us off by covering the science behind why eating the right food is key to fertility and a healthy pregnancy. I'll take you through some common questions about body weight and fertility, nutrient deficiency, and the "epigenetics" of diet and how it can impact fertility, even generations later.

Before we dive into a discussion on which foods to eat (and not eat), chapter 3 covers the basics on nutrition so that you can understand *why* certain foods are recommended for a healthy pregnancy. In this chapter, I'll discuss the key nutrients that women need, especially those closely tied to fertility and pregnancy. For each nutrient, you'll find out how much a woman needs, why she needs it, and which foods provide it. Similar nutritional information will be provided for men in this chapter. Chapter 4 takes you through the psychology of changing habits and the challenges that we all face when trying to change our eating behaviors. This can be challenging, but don't worry, as I have lots of ideas on how to successfully do it! Here you can find practical advice on ways to think about eating in a healthy way, avoid cravings, and cope with the stress that often accompanies trying to conceive (without using food as a way to soothe yourself if you've had a bad day, or reward yourself if you've had a good day).

Next we will jump into part 2 of the book, the Four-Week Fertility-Boosting Plan.

Once you're familiar with the key nutrients and foods associated with fertility and the steps you can take to change eating behaviors, chapter 5 will focus on ways couples can improve fertility with the top twenty specific foods to help boost fertility, and what the research says about these foods (along with some recipes to help). Then, chapter 6 will discuss the research behind the top 20 foods you should avoid when trying to conceive, with alternative healthy options to choose from instead. Chapter 7 will help you to implement the changes in nutrition that we are discussing with additional recipes, meal and snack ideas, and weekly menus to help you plan out your meals. Last but not least, chapter 8 focuses on other things in our food environment aside from the food itself, like chemicals in food packaging, that can impact fertility. Here you'll also find advice on food prep and storage, as well as helpful tips and guidelines to follow when shopping and eating out to ensure that your food is clean, safe, and of course, fertility-friendly.

One final point: Although the focus of this book is on the woman's diet, the role of a man's diet in fertility cannot be overlooked. Thus, throughout the book you will find that there is also information on male fertility and what men can do to boost their sperm health with good nutrition. Making a baby is a team effort, even when it comes to the role that nutrition can play!

Final Thoughts Before We Get Started

Having a baby is a wonderful experience, but getting there isn't always easy. I'd be lying if I told you that changing your diet would *guarantee* you a baby. Unfortunately, that is one guarantee that no one can make. But, you *can* improve your chances of getting pregnant by eating the right foods for the right reasons. I am going to give focused, science-based nutrition advice for *any* woman (or man) who is trying to have a baby: those who are just getting started or thinking of getting started with trying to conceive, those struggling with infertility, and those who might be a while away but want to ensure they are eating healthy for when that time comes. By optimizing nutrition, one can boost fertility, ensure they are creating the best environment for their baby-to-be, and feel good all at the same time.

◆ ◆ ◆

In our modern food environment, it can be hard to eat healthy. With the bombardment of advertisements for delicious foods, easy access to fast-food chains, and those healthier options often being out of reach and harder to come by, most of us struggle to each well on a regular basis. But when you have the added incentive of knowing that the foods you are eating can have a direct impact on your fertility and well-being of your future baby, one's perspective changes. And as you will see throughout this book, it isn't all about discipline or changing your mindset about what you eat. Eating to promote your fertility doesn't have to take much more work, and it doesn't have to cost you an exorbitant amount of money. It still isn't easy, but with the nutritional advice and psychological guidance throughout this book it can be done.

CHAPTER 2

The Importance of Diet for a Healthy Pregnancy

Following a healthy diet is no longer just about achieving an ideal weight or looking a certain way. Eating right is an essential component of treating and preventing a variety of diseases and medical issues. And specifically, nutrition can alter fertility outcomes in both women and men. For example, diets rich in unsaturated fats, whole grains, vegetables, and fish have been shown to positively affect fertility, whereas diets high in saturated fat and/or sugar (also known as a Western diet) may contribute to infertility. I'll go into more details on the specific nutrients that impact fertility (and which foods contain them) in chapter 3, but for now, the take-home point is that what you eat can make a difference for your fertility.

Of course, there are many, many factors that affect fertility. Money, work, stress, depression, body weight, physical activity, substance use, blood pressure, and simply your biological makeup, among many others, can all impact your success in trying to get pregnant and have a baby. But, as I have mentioned earlier, nutrition is one of the things that you can control and change, and by changing your diet to be healthier, you can end up reducing some of these other factors that negatively impact fertility, like high blood pressure and increased body weight.

As I've stated repeatedly, men's health also matters for a healthy pregnancy! In fact, you'll notice that many of the food additives and toxins I talk about throughout the book have more obvious effects on men than women, so nutrition is also an important factor in male fertility.

We'll get into the specific nutrients that are beneficial and detrimental, but for now I want to look at why nutrition matters for a healthy pregnancy, even *before* you get pregnant. In this chapter, I'll first discuss how food-related conditions such as obesity and nutrient deficiency impact your ability to get pregnant. Then, I'll discuss epigenetics and review some of the amazing research on how your nutrition *now* can have an impact on not only your ability to get pregnant but also on your children's (and grandchildren's) health later on.

Why Worry About Weight?

Obesity is on the rise worldwide, so if you happen to be one of the 71.6 percent of Americans (more than 72 million people) who struggle with being overweight or obese, know that you aren't alone. There are many factors that can lead to being overweight or obese. Women (and men) in the Western world have a pretty full plate (no pun intended) of things to deal with. Long work hours, financial stress, and pressure to keep a perfect home and happy family can all lead to less time and energy for focusing on health and fitness. Hectic schedules can result in irregular workout regimens (or even a complete lack of exercise) and less-than-optimal nutrition. Fewer meals are cooked at home, with numerous options for fast and ready-to-eat food. And not only is fast food consumed at high rates, but it is consumed fast; less time devoted to having a meal leads to rushed eating, which in turn can contribute to weight gain as our body's satiety, or fullness response doesn't kick in soon enough to curtail eating. Constant stress can also lead to "stress eating" and overeating, which can add extra pounds. And these are just some of the factors that contribute to overeating and excess weight gain. We haven't even talked about genetics, hormonal imbalances, or ease-of-access to healthier food options.

I am sure you have heard that being overweight or obese can lead to a plethora of health issues, including increased risk of heart disease, cancer, and metabolic syndrome, etc. Further, overweight and obese individuals often suffer from a psychological toll on well-being and happiness. By no means does it mean that if you are overweight or obese you are destined to have health problems; many people who have a body mass index (BMI) that puts them in this category are perfectly happy and healthy. However, you are at higher risk of developing health complications.

I'm not trying to frighten you. Rather, this information is meant to raise awareness about the science regarding the relationship between body weight and fertility and to underscore why it is so important to consider what we are eating when trying to get pregnant. Fortunately, by changing the way you eat now—with help from the rest of the chapters in this book—you may be able to lower this risk.

However, we now know that body weight can also have an impact on fertility. An increasing number of studies show correlations between higher body weight at conception and negative health effects for both the mother and baby. In women, obesity can be linked to reproductive disorders such as polycystic ovary syndrome (PCOS), menstrual disruptions, and decreased effectiveness of fertility treatments. Even for women who are ovulating regularly, the greater the BMI, the longer it seems to take to get pregnant. Women who are overweight or obese at conception have a greater risk for pregnancy complications, including increased risk of miscarriage, gestational diabetes, and high blood pressure (which can lead to dangerous complications called preeclampsia). Obese women also have a higher risk of needing a C-section. There is nothing wrong with needing or getting a C-section, but there are greater risks for infections and complications compared with having a vaginal birth. Also, an overwhelming amount of research shows us that overweight and obesity can cause a variety of reproductive problems in men, not limited to a decline in semen quality, erectile dysfunction, and abnormal reproductive hormone levels. Why does being overweight potentially cause all of these problems? Scientists don't know the exact mechanisms, but it is believed that excess body fat sends signals throughout the body and brain that cause metabolic changes that reduce male and female fertility.

If you are overweight, you might be wondering "If I lose weight, will I regain my fertility?" The good news is that studies suggest that weight loss *can* improve fertility. In women specifically, there is evidence that just a 5 percent weight loss can increase fertility and improve hormonal abnormalities. So if you're a woman who weighs

195 pounds, you will greatly improve your chances of getting pregnant if you lose just under 10 pounds. Further evidence that weight loss can help with fertility comes from research showing improvements in fertility in both men and women who undergo bariatric surgery.

• •

Baby Cleanse?

With the increased popularity of cleanses to "detox" your body from chemicals and impurities, you might be wondering if these are a good idea to try before getting pregnant. My recommendation? Don't do it. Many popular cleanses involve severe calorie restriction or eliminating complete food groups. The truth is, in order to make your body the healthiest it can be, you will need to make healthy changes that involve eating enough calories and having a balanced diet. Any "cleanse" that promises you better health but then tells you to only drink juice for a week is a scam, and if anything, will hurt you in the long run more than it will help you.

• •

Nutrient Deficiency

Most people tend to think that nutrient deficiencies happen to people who live in third-world countries where food is scarce. But the sad reality is that anyone, regardless of weight or access to food, can suffer from nutrient deficiencies. This is especially true in the United States, since even though most people are overweight and have an abundance of food available, the typical Western diet that we consume is full of processed foods that are often devoid of nutrients.

An unbalanced diet, whether lacking micronutrients (like certain vitamins) or macronutrients (like going low-fat or low-carb) can have a negative impact on male and female fertility. An extreme example of this is in women who suffer from eating disorders such as anorexia and bulimia nervosa, in whom we see disruptions in menstrual cycles, higher rates of miscarriage, and generally more difficulty getting pregnant. A similar impact on fertility can be seen in males, although research in males with eating disorders is lacking.

Deficiencies in certain nutrients, which can happen when you don't consume a balanced diet, have been linked to fertility problems. I will cover this in greater detail in chapter 3, but to give you some examples, recent research shows that zinc and selenium deficiencies play a role in infertility. Studies in women with disorders that cause malabsorption, such as celiac disease, have also been shown to have decreased fertility, suggesting that key nutrients such as iron, folic acid, zinc, vitamin B_{12}, and fat-soluble vitamins may all play an important role in reproduction. I'll share a lot more on the specific nutrients that you need, how deficiencies can impact your fertility, and how you can make sure you are eating the right foods to avoid a deficiency from occurring in the next chapter.

So, can eating healthier or addressing deficiencies improve your fertility? Absolutely! Studies show that making the switch to a healthier diet *can* improve fertility outcomes. Some research suggests that dietary supplements could also be helpful when trying to increase fertility. I will talk more about supplements later on, but note that, in most cases, the best thing to do whenever possible is to choose whole foods over processed foods, instead of relying on supplements. Eating a variety of plant and animal foods is key to ensuring you get all the nutrients you need and more.

• •

Keto for Weight Loss When Trying to Conceive?

Many people rave about the wonders of the keto diet for weight loss. You may be wondering: Should I start eating keto to lose some extra weight before getting pregnant? My opinion on this is *no*. While some studies do suggest that the ketogenic diet can help people to lose weight, by cutting out large groups of foods (like fruits and grains) you may be putting yourself at risk for nutrient deficiencies, which can also be harmful to your efforts to conceive. While the keto diet is attractive because people seem to lose weight fast, the reality is that they gain weight back fast, too, when they stop eating that way. And since we don't know much research-wise about the impact of the ketogenic diet on pregnancy, it is not recommended to follow a keto diet when pregnant or trying to get pregnant.

• •

Epigenetics, Nutrition and Your Fertility

Fertility is a lot more than the ability to conceive and carry a baby to term. Both partners' health before conception also influences the future health of a child. Studies show that the diet and lifestyle of both mothers and fathers has *multigenerational* health effects. Let's take a look at some historical examples.

One of the earliest clues that nutrition has a significant, long-term impact on disease outcomes came from the study of people who lived during the Dutch Famine. During the Nazi occupation in 1944–1945, food supply was extremely limited in some parts of the Netherlands. This led to daily food rations as low as 500 calories. The Dutch kept very good records, and later on scientists were able to look at the health information and make some discoveries. In the Dutch Famine Birth Cohort Study, scientists reported the outcome of pregnancies that occurred during this famine period. Results showed a doubled risk of cardiovascular diseases forty to fifty years *later* in those children born to mothers who experienced extremely severe undernutrition during early pregnancy. Also, the serious nutritional deprivation increased the risk of metabolic disorders and breast cancer decades later in this cohort. Notably, depending on the period of starvation (early versus late pregnancy, and pre-conceptional versus postnatal undernutrition) marked differences in disease outcomes were observed.

Another interesting historical epidemiological study pointed out the importance of nutritional status during puberty and its impact on the offspring's health. In the nineteenth century, the Swedish county of Norrbotten was so isolated that if the harvest failed, people starved. Harvest failures caused several famines, and researchers later discovered that if an individual went through a famine as a teenager, his or her *grandchildren* would have a higher mortality risk ratio.

Since these early studies, we have learned a lot more about how nutrition can impact the health of offspring generations later. This is where the field of epigenetics comes in. While these historical accounts focused on nutrient deficiencies as a result of starvation, we now know that life experiences, habits, and our environment shape what and who we are by virtue of their impact on our own personal "epigenome" and health. Behavior, nutrition, and exposure to toxins and pollutants are among the lifestyle factors known to be associated with epigenetic modifications. For example, newer research suggests that the sperm of obese fathers can increase the risk of their offspring becoming obese and having diabetes-like symptoms for up to two generations.

How does this all work? Basically, we all inherit DNA from our parents. Some segments of the DNA, known as genes, can be expressed or not. This means some genes are active, while others are inactive. Studies have shown that factors like diet and lifestyle can influence the expression of genes (i.e., turn them on or off), and as a result we are learning that we are more in control of our destiny (and that of our offspring) than we ever thought possible. Epigenetics is the study of how this expression occurs from our diet, environment, relationships, and stress. A mother's or father's eating habits, exercise regime, stress levels and environment epigenetically have the power to shape the genes passed down and impact the susceptibility of their child to certain health disorders, including but not limited to diabetes, cardiovascular disease, metabolic disorders, cancers, and cognitive function, in later life.

So what does this all mean for you? Well, we can't exactly go back and change our grandmothers' diets or lifestyles, but that doesn't mean that you or your baby are destined to struggle with health problems because of behaviors that might have happened in your family history over fifty years ago. Epigenetics is about turning on and off gene expression. And you can do things, right now, to counteract some of the negative effects on health that you might have inherited. So, even if you aren't looking to get pregnant right now, what you eat is still important. This is one of the many reasons why you should be concerned about your nutrition and health, even before you get pregnant.

◆ ◆ ◆

Now you can see how much of an impact diet can have on fertility, and why paying attention to what you eat can make a difference. In the next chapter, we will look more closely at the various nutrients that you need to stay healthy, how they can play a role in your fertility, and how you can ensure that you are getting enough of them through eating the right foods.

CHAPTER 3

Key Nutrients for Fertility

A growing baby relies entirely on the mother's daily nutrient intake and body stores for healthy growth and development. Their little fingers, toes, eyes, and nose, as well as their nervous system and all other organ systems, are forming and require a continuous supply of "building blocks" for the ongoing "construction." Therefore, consuming nutritious foods is essential to support this growth. So, why am I talking about this when you aren't even pregnant yet? Because, as we discussed in the previous chapter, what you eat before you get pregnant also can have an impact on the baby's development. Plus, we now know from scientific research that diet impacts fertility in many ways, so proper nutrition is essential to helping you get (and stay) pregnant.

Before we get into the plan of which foods you should (and should not) consume when trying to get pregnant, it is important to review some of the basics of nutrition. This way, you will understand *why* certain foods are recommended for promoting a healthy pregnancy, and also be able to recognize healthy nutrients in other foods so that you can make better food choices. In this chapter, I will cover many of the key vitamins, minerals, and nutrients that women (and men) need, with a special emphasis on those nutrients that are tied to fertility and pregnancy. Each of these nutrients will be mentioned further in the rest of the book, so this chapter can serve as a reference section for those who may not be familiar with these not-so-common terms.

Which Nutrients Do You Need?

In this chapter, for each nutrient I will discuss how much a woman needs, why she needs it, and where she can get it from food sources. Similar nutritional information will be provided for the men, too. Note that there are no medically agreed-upon recommended amounts of these nutrients for women who are "trying" to get pregnant, so I have listed the amounts suggested for both nonpregnant and pregnant women, so you can see the differences (many of which are very small).

• •

Food Fact

RDI, RDA, AI and UL. Do all of these abbreviations look like alphabet soup to you? Don't worry, I'll break it all down. **Reference Daily Intake (RDI)** is used to determine the **Daily Value (DV)** of foods, which may be familiar to you from the Nutrition Facts labels (as percent DV) in the United States and Canada. These numbers are regulated by the Food and Drug Administration (FDA) and Health Canada. If a food contains 20 percent or more of a given nutrient's RDI, then "high," "rich in," or "excellent source of" may be used on the label. If the food contains 10–19 percent of the RDI, terms like "good source," "contains," or "provides" can be used on the label.

Recommended Dietary Allowance (RDA) is the average daily level of intake sufficient to meet the nutrient requirements of nearly all (97–98 percent of) healthy people.

Adequate Intake (AI) is the value established when the scientific evidence is not sufficient to develop an RDA. Essentially, this is the "best guess" on how much you need to be healthy, based on what information is available.

Tolerable Upper Intake Level (UL) is maximum daily intake unlikely to cause adverse health effects. You don't want to go beyond the UL for any nutrient where an UL is offered. Doing so can cause serious adverse effects, so it is very important to know about a nutrient's UL whenever possible, especially if you are taking nutritional supplements.

• •

FOLATE/FOLIC ACID (ALSO KNOWN AS VITAMIN B₉)

Women need: 400 micrograms or dietary folate equivalents (DFEs) per day (600 micrograms when pregnant). **Men need:** 400 micrograms. **UL:** 1000 mcg per day

Foods to focus on: spinach, kidney beans, mustard greens, green peas, peanuts, wheat germ, tomato juice, crab, oranges, papaya, and bananas.

Why you need it: You may already be somewhat familiar with this nutrient, as it is recommended for all women of childbearing age regardless of pregnancy status, as well as all men. Folic acid (synthetic form present in supplements or fortified foods), or folate (natural form present in foods) is a B group vitamin (B₉) involved in making and repairing DNA as well as aiding in numerous biological reactions. It is absolutely crucial in cell division, which is why adequate intake is so important early on in pregnancy, when the most rapid growth is occurring with all of those little cells dividing and multiplying. Adequate folate sources are also needed to prevent neural tube defects (such as spina bifida and anencephaly)—the most serious complication of folic acid deficiency, which can cause abnormalities in the baby's brain and spinal cord. The neural tube forms and closes very early on in pregnancy (closure is complete at about four weeks), so daily intake of folate or folic acid *before* conception and during the first month of pregnancy is critical. Further, there is *some* evidence that taking a folic acid supplement before conception and early on in pregnancy can reduce the risk of autism in children, further emphasizing the importance of this vitamin during the very early stages of pregnancy. Lastly, recent research has also shown that women with obesity metabolize folate differently than normal-weight women. Increased body weight has been associated with increased risk for neural tube defects, perhaps because less folate may be available to babies of women with obesity.

Because folate is so critical for cell division, that means that it is important for the cell division of sperm cells, too. Folate levels measured in semen have been associated with sperm count and health. One study found that low folate levels in semen were associated with poor sperm DNA stability, meaning that their viability and overall health may be poor, and this can be a factor in male infertility. Another study found that a combined supplementation of folic acid and zinc (which we will discuss later) for twenty-six weeks increased total sperm count in fertile and subfertile men. In fact, it increased normal total sperm count by 74 percent! This doesn't mean that folic acid is a cure-all for low sperm quality, as in some conditions (like in cases where there are multiple issues related to sperm health, such as shape, motility, and count all being low) it doesn't seem to help, but for many it doesn't hurt to opt for a diet rich in folate-containing foods to help with sperm health.

• •

What Is a DFE?

The reason why folate intake is expressed in DFEs is because food-based folate and folic acid from supplements are not absorbed the same way. One microgram of food-based folate equals 0.6 micrograms of folic acid from supplements or fortified foods if consumed with food and 0.5 micrograms of folic acid if consumed on an empty stomach.

• •

Because natural folate is sensitive to heat, it is best to eat your veggies and fruit fresh and raw, for example as part of a smoothie. However, if you do boil your veggies, grains, or legumes, make sure not to toss out the water, because folate is soluble in water, and that's where it will be. Not sure what to do with that leftover cooking water? Add it to a "green" smoothie, use it as the base of a soup, or mix some into your pasta sauce for an added nutrient boost.

You may be getting folic acid in your diet from foods that don't naturally contain it. This is because the United States started fortifying our food supply with folic acid in 1998 (as did some other countries at varying dates). Folic acid is now present in all white flour and many flour-containing foods such as breads and cereals, which has helped to dramatically reduce the number of babies born with neural tube defects.

So, you may be wondering if you should take a folic acid supplement to help you get pregnant. The current international recommendation is to take a folic acid supplement from the moment you start trying. Most prenatal vitamins contain folic acid or folate, so you should be covered by your prenatal. Men can take a supplement, too. Don't worry—you don't need to convince your partner to take a prenatal vitamin! Stand-alone folic acid supplements are available.

• •

Food Fact

MTHFR. No, it isn't a new curse word abbreviation! MTHFR is an enzyme that makes folic acid usable by the body. Those with a defective MTHFR gene have an impaired ability to produce the MTHFR enzyme. This can make it more difficult to break down and eliminate synthetic folic acid as well as other substances like heavy metals. If you have a mutation of this gene, it means that folic acid can't be converted into usable form, and it can build up in the body. There are also several other nasty symptoms that can emerge, including chronic inflammation, fatigue, allergies, and dizziness. If you find that you do have the mutation, you should use a supplement with methylfolate (not folic acid).

• •

VITAMIN B$_{12}$

Women need: 2.4 micrograms per day (2.6 micrograms when pregnant). **Men need:** 2.4 micrograms per day. **UL:** none established.

Foods to focus on: cooked salmon, broiled beef sirloin, low-fat cow's milk, eggs, clams, trout, chicken breast.

Why you need it: Vitamin B_{12} (also known as cobalamin) can play a big role in fertility. Many people (about 6 percent of the U.S. population) are B_{12} deficient. This can have a host of symptoms, including infertility. Studies show that women who are deficient in B_{12} experience repeated miscarriages and prolonged periods of infertility. Low B_{12} levels might produce changes in the blood that lead to miscarriage as well as changes that contribute to abnormal ovulation, impaired development of the egg, and difficulty implanting a fertilized egg. The good news is that increasing B_{12} levels can, in some cases, correct ovulation and improve fertility. B_{12} is closely related to folate and is crucial for brain and nervous system development, blood formation, and numerous other reactions that take place in just about every cell of a baby's growing body. Similar to folic acid, being deficient in B_{12} can increase the risk of neural tube defects. Research shows that low levels of B_{12} very early in pregnancy increase the risk of neural tube defects nearly threefold, whereas adequate intake of B_{12} has a protective effect against these defects. In fact, taking a daily B_{12} supplement in addition to folic acid at least three months before conception and for the first three months of pregnancy—if you are or may be vitamin B_{12} deficient—may also prevent the risk of neural tube defects better than taking folic acid alone. There is a biochemical explanation for this: Without adequate levels of B_{12}, folate can't be metabolized appropriately and used by the cells.

· ·

Food Fact

Vitamin B_{12} is only found in animal products, which is why it is of particular importance if you are vegan or vegetarian, as you may be lacking the vitamin in your diet (in which case you should consult your physician and may need to take vitamin B_{12} supplements or shots).

· ·

For men, there is also a link between vitamin B_{12} levels and infertility. B_{12} plays an important part in the production and development of sperm. By extension, when you are deficient in or have low levels of B_{12}, it can take a toll on your sperm health. Studies show a link between a lower concentration of plasma vitamin B_{12} and infertility in men. B_{12} supplementation has shown promise and is, in fact, recommended when sperm count is affected. One study found that when 1500 mcg of methylcobalamin, a form of vitamin B_{12}, was administered daily to infertile men for a period ranging from four to twenty-four weeks, the total sperm count increased in 53.8 percent of cases and sperm concentration increased in 38.4 percent of cases.

ZINC

Women need: 8 milligrams per day (11 milligrams per day when pregnant). *Men need:* 11 mg per day. *UL:* 40 milligrams per day.

Foods to focus on: Alaskan king crab, canned baked beans, fortified breakfast cereals, lamb, turkey, tofu, pumpkin seeds, garbanzo beans, wheat germ, yogurt, milk, and collard greens.

Why you need it: Zinc is a basic element that makes up genetic material, and if there is a deficit in the body, this will clearly affect fertility. Zinc is needed for rapidly dividing cells and protein and DNA synthesis as well as for numerous other reactions that take place when a baby is trying to develop. In women, zinc helps the body use the sexual hormones (e.g., progesterone) efficiently, and it is required for the production of healthy eggs. Zinc is also an element that supports the health of the immune system, which needs to be in tip-top shape when trying to get pregnant.

Similarly, in men, zinc is important for the body to be able to utilize the male sexual hormones and estrogen in an efficient manner. Zinc is normally found in the composition of the sperm. It makes up the coating and the tail of the sperm, and if there is a deficiency of zinc in the system, the quality of the sperm will be inferior. Zinc also influences sperm count. Studies show that men with a reduced zinc intake also tend to have a reduced sperm count. Zinc also plays a role in testosterone synthesis, prostate health, and fertilization.

Even if you don't have symptoms of zinc deficiency (such as suppressed appetite, growth retardation, and reduced immune function, which are often only present in severe deficiency), you may still be consuming less zinc than recommended. Besides food sources, you can also get this element from zinc supplements. Look for zinc acetate or zinc picolinate or zinc citrate, as these are the best-tolerated and most bioavailable forms of zinc in a supplement form. Stay clear of zinc oxide (the stuff in sunblock!), as it's the least absorbent form of zinc. Lastly, it is important to constantly get zinc in your system (either by eating zinc-rich foods or by taking zinc supplements), because the body can't store it.

• •

Food Fact

We absorb less zinc from non-animal sources, which may be a concern if you're vegan or vegetarian. However, you can increase the amount of zinc you absorb by soaking and cooking legumes and combining plant-based zinc sources with acidic ingredients such as lemon juice.

• •

VITAMIN B_6

Women need: 1.3 milligrams per day (1.9 milligrams per day when pregnant). **Men need:** 1.3 milligrams per day. **UL:** 100 milligrams per day.

Foods to focus on: baked potato, salmon, chicken, cooked spinach, prune juice, chickpeas, brown rice, banana, avocado, pork loin.

Why you need it: Vitamin B_6, otherwise known as pyridoxine, is another important B vitamin that helps your body metabolize macronutrients such as proteins, carbohydrates, and fat. It also helps to form new red blood cells, is involved in brain and nervous system development by making neurotransmitters (brain chemicals), and participates in numerous other reactions. Research also shows that adequate vitamin B_6 levels before conception and early in pregnancy may help to prevent pregnancy loss. Also, being B_6 deficient is linked to irregular menstrual cycles, progesterone imbalance, poor egg health, and premenstrual syndrome. For men, lack of vitamin B_6 has been linked to poor sperm health.

• •

Food Fact

B vitamins are water-soluble, meaning that what you don't use will be excreted. So, just one day of eating well to increase your B_6 consumption isn't going to cut it. Also, up to 90 percent of the vitamin can be destroyed in the processing of food (cooking, steaming, etc.), so try to eat raw forms of foods, when reasonable.

• •

If you're taking a prenatal vitamin, it likely has 100 percent of the daily dose of B_6, which, in addition to the many vitamin B_6-rich foods that you may be consuming as part of your normal diet, provides you with a more than adequate daily dose of the vitamin. A mild excess of B_6 is unlikely to cause any negative effects. However, it is important to note that there is an upper limit for vitamin B_6 of 100 mg/day, so don't overdo it.

MAGNESIUM

Women need: If you are 19–30 years old: 310 milligrams per day (350 milligrams per day during pregnancy). If you are 31–50 years old: 320 milligrams per day (360 milligrams per day during pregnancy). **Men need:** If you are 19–30 years old: 400 milligrams per day. If you are 31–50 years old: 420 milligrams per day. **UL:** 350 milligrams per day for women and men, from supplements only; food sources don't count.

Foods to focus on: Pumpkin and sunflower seeds, salmon, halibut, wheat germ, bran cereal, quinoa, brown rice, almonds, cashews, spinach, tofu, baked potato (with skin), and yogurt.

Why you need it: Magnesium is an important mineral that serves several different functions. It helps to keep bones healthy, and it also regulates blood sugar levels, muscle and nerve functioning, blood pressure, and making DNA. When it comes to fertility, magnesium is important because it supports progesterone production and increases the blood supply to the uterus, as well as being important for healthy egg production. One study found that among women who had recently discontinued using contraception in an effort to get pregnant, those who had more magnesium in their diets showed a 51.5 percent higher probability of becoming pregnant. Research also shows that magnesium, when taken along with another mineral that we will talk about soon, selenium, helps lower the risk of miscarriage. Magnesium supplements might not be for you if you have certain health conditions. It is always good to speak with your doctor before taking any supplement, but in this case, if you have heart or kidney disease magnesium supplementation might not be recommended.

Magnesium is important for male fertility, too. Magnesium is an essential component of sperm production and function. Studies have found that a reduction of magnesium concentration in seminal fluid may lead to male infertility.

IRON

Women need: 18 milligrams per day (27 milligrams per day when pregnant). **Men need:** 8 milligrams per day. **UL:** 45 milligrams per day.

Foods to focus on: breakfast cereal (fortified with 100 percent DV of iron), spinach, baked potato with skin, firm tofu, and oil-roasted cashew nuts.

Why you need it: Iron helps your body make hemoglobin, which is needed for your blood to carry oxygen. It is also needed for supplying your muscles with oxygen and maintaining a healthy immune system. When it comes to fertility, it seems that iron can have a role. In one study, researchers found that women who took iron supplements had a significantly lower risk of ovulatory infertility (an inability to produce healthy baby-making eggs) than those who didn't take the supplement. Does that mean you need to take a supplement? Not necessarily. More research is needed before I would recommend iron supplements to *all* women as a fertility booster, but even if iron isn't recommended to improve fertility for you specifically, you'll still want to beef up your iron stores the natural way before you get pregnant. Iron is one of the minerals that your future baby-to-be will siphon from you—and too little iron at the start of pregnancy can put you at risk for anemia during pregnancy and afterward (when you need all the energy you can get to take care of your baby).

• •

Food Fact

Not all iron is the same. There are two types of iron—heme and nonheme iron. Heme iron comes only from animal foods, such as meats and organ meats (especially liver), fish, seafood (like clams), and poultry. It is the better-absorbed form of iron, with an approximately 15 to 35 percent absorption rate. Nonheme iron exists in both animal and plant foods and is found in fortified cereals, eggs, milk, pumpkin seeds, lentils and other legumes, spinach, and prune juice. However, the majority of the iron in these foods is poorly absorbed. Not to worry, though! You can bump up your nonheme iron absorption by eating foods rich in vitamin C alongside the nonheme iron sources, such as having lentils with red bell peppers, or indulging in a fresh fruit dessert after a legume meal—strawberries, papayas, kiwi, oranges, cantaloupe, and guava are all packed with vitamin C!

• •

Iron supplements are known to induce nausea. If you're taking a supplement to get your iron, but it makes you so nauseous that you can't eat anything else, then it's worth considering the risks and benefits associated with the consumption of one nutrient versus a deficiency of many more. Because of these concerns, it may be a good idea to first get your blood iron (serum ferritin) levels checked out, and then follow your doctor's advice regarding iron supplementation depending on your iron levels.

● ●

Food Fact

Certain foods can up your nonheme iron absorption, whereas others will prevent your gut from taking in whatever little iron there is in a given bean, veggie, or other nonheme iron source. Here are some examples of absorption enhancers and inhibitors to make sure you can get the most out of what you eat.

Absorption enhancers:

- Vitamin C—can nearly triple the rate of absorption
- Heme-iron sources such as meats, fish, and seafood

Absorption inhibitors:

- Phytic acid that is present in plant foods (such as grains and legumes)
- Fiber
- Coffee and tea (tannic acid in tea)
- Calcium, zinc, magnesium, copper
- Egg protein (in whites and in yolk)
- Some herbs. If you're an avid tea drinker, make sure to moderate your intake of chamomile, peppermint, feverfew and St. John's wort as they can lower your iron absorption rate. If you're unsure about a certain herb, always consult your doctor.

● ●

OMEGA-3 FATTY ACIDS: EPA, DHA, AND ALA

Women need: 1100 milligrams per day of omega-3s; 1400 milligrams per day of omega-3 fatty acids per day, of which 300 milligrams or more are from DHA, when pregnant. **Men need:**1600 milligrams of omega-3s per day. **UL:** not established.

Foods to focus on: salmon, catfish, canned light tuna, anchovies, herring, halibut, fish oil, DHA-enriched eggs, purified fish and algal supplements, and fortified milk and yogurt.

Why you need it: Finally—the popular omega-3s you may have been wondering about while reading about all the other nutrients that are important for growing a healthy baby. Several different omega-3s exist, but the majority of scientific research focuses on three: alpha-linolenic acid (ALA), eicosapentaenoic acid (EPA), and docosahexaenoic acid (DHA). ALA is considered an essential fatty acid, meaning that it must be obtained from the diet. ALA can be converted into EPA and then to DHA, but the conversion (which occurs primarily in the liver) is very limited, with reported rates of less than 15 percent. Therefore, consuming EPA and DHA directly from foods and/or dietary supplements is the only practical way to increase levels of these fatty acids in the body. Numerous studies show health benefits of consuming EPA and DHA, with higher intakes associated with healthy brain development and improved memory as well as improved cognitive and intellectual abilities in childhood and later in life.

When it comes to fertility, increasing your intake of omega-3s seems to be able to help. One research study (conducted in mice) found that a long-term consumption of a diet rich in omega-3 fatty acids could prolong reproductive function into an advanced maternal age. This study also found that a short-term treatment of omega-3 fatty acids could help improve egg (oocyte) quality.

For men, boosting omega-3 intake can help with sperm quality. DHA fatty acids have been found in high concentrations in sperm, suggesting that the DHA molecules are important for their viability, maturity, and functional characteristics. In addition, studies have found that higher levels of omega-3s correlate with improved sperm morphology and motility.

So how do you get the right amount of DHA and EPA? Fortunately, many foods that contain DHA often also have EPA—so that makes things a bit easier. While certain foods, such as eggs, juice, and milk, are fortified with omega-3s, the general recommendation is to consume fatty fish at least twice a week (up to 12 ounces)—from safe food sources (i.e., fish low in mercury, with less than 0.05 parts per billion of mercury in one serving of fish). However, it may still be difficult to get the recommended amount of DHA and EPA from fortified foods and the recommended two servings of fish/seafood per week. Two weekly servings of fish provide only about 100 to 250 mg of omega-3 fatty acids per day (although amounts vary—some fish, such as salmon, have much more EPA and DHA than others), of which 50 to 100 mg is from DHA. Even if you add in plant-based oils, since they supply only miniscule amounts of EPA and no DHA, you're still at a total EPA and DHA amount that is much lower than recommended. It may therefore be a good idea to consider adding a supplement to your diet. In addition, if you're vegan/vegetarian, you very likely need to supplement your diet in order to provide adequate amounts of EPA and DHA to support healthy brain development of a baby, as your diet is naturally lacking them. However, it is still unclear whether enough EPA and DHA can be made by your body if you have an adequate intake of ALA—another major omega-3 fatty acid that is found in plants, such as nuts, oils, and certain greens.

• •

Food Fact

Even though fatty fish are great sources of DHA and other omega-3 fatty acids, it may be a good idea to alternate between eating fish, fortified eggs, and algae, and consider taking a supplement to make sure that you get all the DHA you need. I say this because pollutants found in fish, such as mercury and PBAs, are not helpful for fertility. I'll discuss this more in chapter 8, but, for now, keep in mind that it's best to stick with salmon (wild-caught), sardines, herring, trout, Atlantic and Pacific mackerel, anchovies, canned light tuna, shrimp, pollack, and catfish. See page 122 for a list of fish that are low and high in mercury content.

• •

CALCIUM

Women need: 1,000 milligrams per day (same when pregnant). ***Men need:*** 1,000 milligrams per day. ***UL:*** 2,500 milligrams per day.

Foods to focus on: Many commonly consumed foods—both dairy and nondairy—are good sources of calcium. Dairy sources include milk, yogurt, natural and processed cheeses, cottage cheese, and ice cream. Great nondairy sources are calcium-fortified orange juice, calcium-set tofu, kale, collard greens, broccoli, sardines, dried peas and beans, and roasted almonds.

Why you need it: The majority of American women don't consume enough calcium in their diet, which is why it's so important to focus on adequate calcium intake at this time. However, taking in too much calcium can cause constipation (main side effect of too much calcium) and decrease your absorption of magnesium, so remember that more is not always better.

When it comes to fertility, calcium has a big role. Minerals like calcium help to create an alkaline environment in the reproductive tract, and this is needed to move the sperm toward the egg. Also, one study found that calcium is a vital ingredient in the process of triggering growth in embryos, so it's important for there to be adequate calcium in the surrounding fluid.

Food Fact

Even though there are many sources of calcium, a good old glass of milk (as well as plain yogurt) provides the most calcium per a single serving. Fortified tofu is a close second, whereas to get the same amount of calcium from greens (turnip, Chinese cabbage, mustard greens, kale) and broccoli will require you to consume two to five servings. Lastly, even though spinach is abundant in calcium, the calcium is not bioavailable because it contains oxalic acid, which prevents your body from absorbing it. (However, spinach is a great source of other nutrients, so you should not avoid it, by any means!)

VITAMIN D

Women need: 15 micrograms (600 IUs) per day (same when pregnant). **Men need:** 15 micrograms (600 IUs) per day. **UL:** 100 micrograms (4000 IUs).

Foods to focus on: sockeye salmon, vitamin D–fortified orange juice (the amounts vary depending on the brand), eggs (note that vitamin D is only in the yolk).

Why you need it: Also known as the "sunshine vitamin" because it can be made by your body upon exposure to sunlight, vitamin D helps to maintain adequate levels of calcium and phosphorus, which are especially important for fertility and a healthy pregnancy.

If you are trying to conceive, it is important to pay attention to the amount of vitamin D you are getting in your diet. The active form of vitamin D (calcitriol) has many roles in female reproduction. Calcitriol is able to control the genes involved in making estrogen, which is needed for pregnancy. The uterine lining produces calcitriol in response to the embryo as it enters the uterine cavity, shortly before implantation. Calcitriol controls several genes involved in embryo implantation. Once a woman becomes pregnant, the uterus and placenta continue to make calcitriol, which helps organize immune cells in the uterus so that infections can be fought without harming the pregnancy. Poor vitamin D status has been associated with certain pregnancy complications, such as hypertension and diabetes.

It is also important for men to be mindful of their vitamin D status, as studies suggests it plays an important role in their reproductive health. In fact, vitamin D status has been linked not only to fertility but also to sexual function and testosterone levels. Vitamin D deficiency is more prevalent among men with low semen production, quality, and motility.

• •

What Are the Best Sources of Vitamin D?

The best sources of vitamin D are animal products such as fatty fish (salmon, canned tuna, canned sardines, and catfish) and eggs, as well as fortified foods such as milk, orange juice, margarine, and cereal. However, when choosing the latter foods, make sure to read the label, as not all of them will be fortified (e.g., some margarines are not fortified), and go for the ones that have added vitamin D to get more of it in your diet. In addition, and especially if you don't live in a place with year-round sunshine, a vitamin D supplement may be beneficial. You should speak to your doctor regarding the exact dosage to aim for, because, based on current research, an optimal safe dose has not yet been established, even though the overall conclusion based on vitamin D supplementation research is that supplementing is beneficial.

• •

POTASSIUM

Women need: 2600 milligrams per day (2900 milligrams per day when pregnant). **Men need:** 3400 milligrams per day. **UL:** not established.

Foods to Focus on: sweet potato baked in skin, baked winter squash, lentils, raw kale, fresh fruits (like bananas) and vegetables, fruit and vegetable juices (carrot, prune, tomato), fish (like halibut or coho), nuts, seeds, dried fruits, beans, and milk and other dairy products.

Why you need it: Potassium is a key mineral that helps you maintain optimal electrolyte and fluid balance in all your cells. In addition, potassium is involved in muscle contraction and brain and nerve function. When it comes to your fertility, potassium is important, particularly for men. A deficiency in potassium, known as hypokalemia, can have a significant effect on the health of a man's seminal fluids. Interestingly, there is a link between sodium and potassium that can make it difficult to have the proper balance of these nutrients. The more sodium that one consumes, the more potassium the body will excrete. This makes people who sweat profusely or exercise often at risk for a drop in potassium and an overall drop in fertility. Does this mean that if you are trying to get pregnant you should stop working out? Not at all! But it does mean that you should be extra mindful of staying hydrated and keeping sodium intake low.

VITAMIN A

Women need: 700 micrograms RAE (retinol activity equivalents) (770 micrograms RAE during pregnancy). ***Men need***: 900 micrograms RAE. ***UL***: 3,000 micrograms RAE.

Foods to focus on: raw kale, carrots, eggs, sweet potato baked in skin, oatmeal, cantaloupe, spinach, and cheese

Why you need it: Vitamin A is involved in fat metabolism and tissue repair. Vitamin A is also essential for healthy development of a baby's organs (heart, lungs, brain, kidneys, bones, nerves, eyes) during the embryonic period, and most of this period will occur *before* you know you are pregnant, so it is best to eat accordingly just in case. For men, vitamin A plays a role in sperm health. Men with a diet low in vitamin A are at risk for having their sperm cells stick together instead of them acting individually. When this happens, the sperm cells are inhibited and cannot reach the egg. Think of it like trying to run a race tied to 10,000 other people. Odds are, you all won't be moving so swiftly.

• •

Food Fact

Vitamin A exists in two forms: preformed vitamin A, or retinol, which is found in animal sources, and provitamin A, or carotenoids (the main one of which is beta-carotene), which are found in plant sources and get converted to retinol in the body. It is important to understand this difference. Too much carotene will not harm you, whereas an excess of retinol can lead to liver toxicity and fetal abnormalities. In addition, the average intake of vitamin A in the United States is typically adequate, because preformed vitamin A is abundant in many animal foods, and numerous plant foods contain lots of provitamin A. Therefore, it is unnecessary and often not recommended to take a vitamin A supplement, especially if the supplement contains the preformed vitamin A, in order to avoid the risks of fetal abnormalities and liver toxicity.

You don't have to worry about your carotenoid intake (and some veggies, such as sweet potato, can be very high in it), but do limit your intake of animal foods that have tons of the preformed vitamin A, such as liver, in order to prevent any detrimental consequences of taking in too much vitamin A. I doubt that liver will fall high on your list of most-craved foods, but if it does, I would advise avoiding liver completely if you are trying to get pregnant, because its vitamin A concentration is so high that eating even a couple bites can put you way over your daily recommendation for vitamin A intake (and can even exceed the safe upper limit of vitamin A intake). Finally, know that retinol and beta-carotene are not equal in terms of the potency of vitamin A—it takes twelve times more beta-carotene (provitamin A) to equal 1 microgram of retinol, or preformed vitamin A.

● ●

VITAMIN C

Women need: 75 milligrams per day (85 mg during pregnancy). **Men need:** 90 milligrams per day. **UL:** 2000 milligrams per day.

Foods to focus on: Many fresh fruits and vegetables (especially citrus fruits and leafy greens) contain vitamin C, such as oranges, broccoli, guava, papaya, bell peppers (yellow, green, red), sweet potato, mango, and brussels sprouts. Vitamin C is easily lost during cooking, so raw fruits and vegetables are your best bet.

Why you need it: Vitamin C, or ascorbic acid, is an antioxidant that protects your cells from oxidative damage. It also helps your body fight infections, heal wounds, and repair tissues, and it is involved in collagen synthesis, thus helping to maintain healthy skin. Collagen isn't just for fixing wrinkles! In fact, it is crucial for a developing baby, as collagen is a structural component of connective tissues such as tendons, cartilage, blood vessels, bone matrix, and cornea, making adequate vitamin C intake essential for healthy growth and development.

Vitamin C is important for fertility in women, especially if their progesterone levels are low. One study found that when women with low progesterone took 750 mg of vitamin C per day, 77 percent of those women saw an increase in progesterone levels, leading to an increased rate of pregnancy (25 percent); rate of pregnancy was only 11 percent among women with no treatment. The study also found that vitamin C supplementation resulted in 53 percent of women with luteal phase defect (which is characterized by having low progesterone levels, making pregnancy unlikely) experiencing a lengthening of their luteal phase (and those trying to conceive became pregnant).

Vitamin C is also an important component of sperm health. One study showed that increasing the daily amount of vitamin C in men helps them produce more sperm, stronger sperm, and more mobile sperm. In some cases, the sperm count even rose to be over ten times the amount it was prior to when the men started ingesting a healthy amount of vitamin C. Another study found that supplementation of 1000 milligrams of vitamin C twice daily for a maximum of 2 months increased sperm count and motility. How does vitamin C work to promote sperm health? Since vitamin C is an antioxidant, it is thought to help protect sperm and their DNA from damage. And you want healthy sperm, as the damaged ones fail to thrive at all, fail to allow for conception, or if they do make it to the egg can cause birth defects or a failure for an embryo or fetus to thrive.

Should You Take a Collagen Supplement?

Collagen supplements have become quite popular, and are touted as being a great protein source, having beauty benefits and possibly helping with weight loss. But should you take a collagen supplement if you are trying to get pregnant? As of now, there aren't any studies suggesting that collagen will help promote fertility, or harm it, so it is hard to gauge. Some doctors suggest that it is safe to use while pregnant, and can even help to minimize the stretch marks and hair loss that sometimes comes after the baby is born, but there are few, if any, clinical studies to suggest that these claims are true. My advice? Skip it if you are trying to conceive until we know more, and instead focus on getting your protein and other nutrients from whole foods that we know will have the added bonus of helping to promote fertility.

● ●

SELENIUM

Women need: 55 micrograms per day (60 micrograms per day during pregnancy). **Men need:** 55 micrograms per day. **UL:** 400 micrograms per day.

Foods to focus on: Brazil nuts, roasted ham, sardines, halibut, shrimp, macaroni, roasted turkey, eggs, whole wheat bread, and spinach.

Why you need it: Selenium can be helpful in lowering some autoimmune antibodies, making it an important nutrient for overall immune function. It also seems to play a key role in fertility.

One study found that selenium is crucial to the development of healthy ovarian follicles (remember, follicles are responsible for the production of eggs in women). Another study found that recurrent miscarriage was associated with low selenium levels (the selenium levels were collected via hair samples).

For men, selenium is also important for fertility. Selenium is needed to maintain the shape of sperm mitochondria (which is basically the energy source for the sperm). Also, another important function of selenium is that it protects fatty acids from oxidizing (which is a bad thing). Sperm are mainly made of essential fatty acids, and selenium helps to make sure they don't get destroyed.

Selenium is found in a variety of foods, so supplementation isn't typically necessary. Keep in mind that selenium at higher doses can be toxic, and it is recommended that the daily intake of selenium should not exceed 400 mcg (micrograms, not milligrams) per day, from all sources, including food and supplements.

. . . .

What About the Other Vitamins and Minerals?

In this chapter, we only discussed those nutrients that studies suggest have a role in fertility. Some, like phosphorus, copper, and vitamin E, we didn't touch upon. That doesn't mean that you don't need them for a healthy diet or pregnancy; it is just likely if you are eating a variety of foods you will get them by default.

. . . .

Nutrient	Daily recommended amount for women	Daily recommended amount for men	Dietary sources
Folate/folic acid (Vitamin B_9)	400 micrograms or DFEs (600 when pregnant)	400 micrograms	Spinach, kidney beans mustand greens, green peas, peanuts, wheat germ, tomato juice, crab, oranges, papaya, bananas
Vitamin B_{12}	2.4 micrograms (2.6 when pregnant)	2.4 micrograms	Cooked salmon, low-fat cow's milk, eggs, beef, chicken
Zinc	8 milligrams (11 when pregnant)	11 milligrams	Alaskan King crab, baked beans, fortified breakfast cereal, turkey, tofu, chickpeas, pumpkin seeds, yogurt
Vitamin B_6	1.3 milligrams (1.9 when pregnant)	1.3 milligrams	Baked potato, salmon, chicken, cooked spinach, chickpeas, banana, avocado, brown rice
Magnesium	19–30 years old: 310 milligrams (350 milligrams during pregnancy) 31–50 years old: 320 milligrams (360 when pregnant)	19–30 years old: 400 milligrams 31–50 years old: 420 milligrams	Pumpkin and sunflower seeds, salmon, bran cereal, quinoa, brown rice, almonds, cashews, spinach, tofu, yogurt

Nutrient	Daily recommended amount for women	Daily recommended amount for men	Dietary sources
Iron	18 milligrams (27 when pregnant)	8 milligrams	Fortified breakfast cereal, spinach, tofu, oil roasted cashew nuts
Omega-3 fatty acids (EPA, DHA, ALA)	1400 milligrams (300+ must come from DHA when pregnant)	1600 milligrams	Salmon, catfish, tuna, anchovies, fish oil, DHA-enriched eggs, fortified milk and yogurt
Calcium	1000 milligrams	1000 milligrams	Milk, yogurt, cheeses, calcium-fortified orange juice, kale, broccoli, sardines, roasted almonds
Vitamin D	15 micrograms	15 micrograms	Sockeye salmon, vitamin-D fortified orange juice, eggs
Potassium	2600 milligrams (2900 when pregnant)	3400 milligrams	Sweet potato and winter squash baked in skin, lentils, kale, banana, halibut, salmon, nuts, seeds, dried fruits, dairy products
Vitamin A	700 micrograms RAE (retinol activity equivalents) (770 microgram RAE when pregnant)	900 micrograms RAE	Kale, carrots, eggs, sweet potato, melon, spinach, cheese
Vitamin C	75 milligrams (85 when pregnant)	90 milligrams	Many fresh fruits and vegetables (especially citrus and leafy greens)
Selenium	55 micrograms (60 when pregnant)	55 micrograms	Brazil nuts, roasted ham, sardines, halibut, shrimp, eggs, whole wheat bread, spinach

◆ ◆ ◆

Whew! That was a lot of information, but I bet you now know more than you ever thought you would about nutrition in fertility. So, now that we have covered the key nutrients that can promote your fertility, *why* they are key, and *where* you can find them, we can begin to delve into part 2 of the book. The chapters in part 2 are designed to outline my Four-Week Fertility-Boosting Plan and help you to identify foods that you should try to incorporate into your diet (or cut out of your diet) to help ensure that you are using good nutrition to your advantage when it comes to your fertility.

This certainly doesn't mean that you need to eat *all* of the foods discussed here or in the next section every day (or even every week) to boost your fertility! Remember that most foods you consume contain multiple nutrients. For example, cooked lentils contain folate, iron, fiber, phosphorus, protein, vitamins B_1 and B_6, potassium, and zinc, among other nutrients, helping you get part of your daily dose of all of these nutrients. The goal here is to try to eat foods that are healthy, wholesome, and contain nutrients that we know will be beneficial to you and your fertility. Plus, the four-week guide will help you to make eating healthy manageable, and maybe even fun, because you can be thinking of how the great food you are eating and recipes you can try out are helping you get one step closer to getting pregnant!

PART II:

The Four-Week Fertility-Boosting Nutrition Plan

CHAPTER 4

The Psychology of Eating Behaviors

Now that you are armed with all of the background information on fertility and nutrition, we can get to the fun part. This Four-Week Fertility-Boosting Plan is pretty simple: you can take control over your diet and make changes to your eating behaviors by incorporating more fertility-promoting foods and cutting back on those foods that can be detrimental to fertility. I am going to provide you with meal ideas, recipes, and menus to help. While this plan sounds simple, enacting it might not be so easy for some of us. This is because of the power of habit and how hard it can be to break unhealthy eating behaviors—even when you are highly motivated to make a change. But don't worry, because in this chapter we are going to go over some ways you can psychologically and emotionally change your relationship with food, for the better.

As someone who works in the field of psychology and nutrition, one of the things that frustrates me most is when someone *talks* about a diet or eating plan and just leaves it at that. Changing your eating habits is a lot more than just shopping lists and recipes. Anyone can order groceries or cook a meal, but the challenge comes in sustaining these behaviors and making changes that you can stick to (and not feel like you are depriving yourself). That's where the psychology comes in. You will see that the Four-Week Fertility-Boosting Plan includes not only suggestions on what to eat but also practical and psychological mini-tasks and tips to help you redevelop your relationship with food. For some of us, changing eating habits might be relatively easy to do, but for others it can take some more time to get things to stick, and also require some support along the way.

This chapter will focus on the psychology of changing habits and the challenges that we all face when trying to change our eating behaviors. Practical advice on ways to think about eating in a healthy way, avoiding cravings, and not self-medicating with food will be discussed in detail so you can start working on changing your habits to be healthy ones now.

The Power of Habits

Let's take a step back for a second and talk about how we form habits in the first place. Habits are nothing more than learning to the extreme. When we learn an association between two things, and that association is repeated over and over again, the association gets stronger. At some point, these associations become so strong that we don't even need to think about them; the behavior automatically happens without even thinking about it. For example, think about putting on your seat belt when you get in the car. You most likely do this reflexively and don't need to remind yourself to buckle up when you get in. It just happens because you do it so often.

Let's look at another example. Let's say you decide to start taking your niece out for ice cream on Fridays after she finishes school. The first time you take her, she will no doubt be very happy and the action triggers her "reward" center in the brain. Because your niece loves ice cream (and you!), the Friday-afternoon treat is rewarding, and will continue to be so even after it becomes habitual (because you go every week) and is no longer a special event. This is because the brain's reward center (which releases dopamine, a neurotransmitter that plays a role in how we feel pleasure) continues to be stimulated even after something becomes a habit. This effect of habit and rewarding experiences can be advantageous to our health goals. For example, this is why habitual exercise can be rewarding (the runner's "high" comes from the rush of dopamine and brain opioids).

Habits are a normal part of everyday life and are typically useful—for example, eating breakfast when you wake up, hanging your keys on a hook by the door when you come home, or brushing your teeth before going to bed. However, when our reward system is involved, repetitive behaviors (especially those that make you feel good) can be extremely hard to change. Dopamine is basically like adding an extra layer of reinforcement to the behavior, which is why it becomes harder to break. This can be a good thing, but when unhealthy behaviors are reinforced, it can be detrimental to our health in the long run. Many of the habits that we are trying to break are unhealthy ones, and these habits, much like putting on our seat belt, may be so automatic that we don't even notice them until we take a step back. Snacking on sweets whenever you're feeling tired, mindlessly eating when watching TV, or having a glass of wine (or two) as soon as you get home from work are some examples of habits that you might not even realize you have developed.

Food Makes Me Happy

It's no secret that our emotions and our eating habits are closely intertwined. Whether we're sad, happy, stressed, anxious, or excited, our emotions can have an impact on when, what, and how much we eat and vice versa. We often seek food to get immediate satisfaction, or in some cases, relief (see self-medicating section below), and this usually works. Typically, these types of foods tend to be what we call "comfort foods." Comfort foods could really be any type of food, but more often than not they include things high in fat and/or sugar like potato chips, fried foods, soda, breads and pastas, candy, or pastries.

Although these comfort foods tend to make us happy while we are eating them, fruits and vegetables are what will actually make a lasting impression on your mood. Researchers are finding that increasing your consumption of healthier foods, like fruits and vegetables, is more likely to increase your happiness and life satisfaction in the long run versus the sweets. On the other hand, eating a Western diet (a diet high in fat, sugar, and salt, i.e. sugary beverages, processed meats, fried foods, and baked goods) is associated with the onset, maintenance, and severity of depressive symptoms and disorders. Knowing this, it will probably come as no surprise to you that eating more fruits and vegetables may also improve symptoms or decrease risk of depression.

That's not to say that fruits and vegetables can't make you happy in the moment, either. A study conducted in 2017 compared in-the-moment psychological benefits of eating foods in fourteen different categories, one being vegetables, with others like grains, sweets, fruits, and dairy. The researchers found that fruits and vegetables can have an immediate mood-boosting effect similar to that of sweets. In fact, they did not find a significant difference in feelings between the two (and both categories produced the highest mood-boosting effects). So although eating something unhealthy may be associated with tastiness, and thus we immediately feel good when we eat it (thanks to the dopamine rush from our brain reward center), it's possible that eating things like fruits and vegetables can boost our mood because of the health factor—we feel happy that we are eating something healthy that we know is good for us. Or is could be that our bodies detect all of the great nutrients in fruits and veggies and the happy signal gets sent to our brain as a result.

Despite these findings, it's clear that we seem to be drawn more to less-healthy foods, especially when we're not feeling our best. Self-medicating with food is extremely common, and despite the benefits associated with healthy foods, we still tend to "heal" ourselves with less-healthy ones. Let's take a look at why this happens and ways that you can try to make better choices the next time you are tempted to do it.

Self-Medicating with Food

Think about the last time you were not feeling so happy. I bet you didn't go and eat a big salad to make yourself feel better. You probably opted for something sweet, like cookies or ice cream, or full of fat like chips or buttery mashed potatoes, to help boost your spirits. And, it probably worked.

Although there are a variety of emotions that could lead us to self-medicate with food, stress is arguably one of the biggest contributors. Of course, everyone has a different response to stress, but research shows that "everyday" stress is more likely to cause people to overeat. The overeating caused by these small, daily stressors, which are sometimes referred to as "daily hassles" (think traffic, having ten loads of laundry to do, or holiday family stress) usually includes energy-dense, sugar-rich food. In fact, research shows that a "binge" on palatable and energy-dense foods such as sweets, breads, or pastas can actually reduce feelings of anger or tension and increase a sense of calmness within 1–2 hours of eating. (This is not unlike what we see with drug addiction; the self-medicating behavior of resorting to drug use in times of stress or not feeling great is comparable to what we see in binge-eating behavior.) The majority of people who eat (especially unhealthy foods) when they're stressed say it is because the food makes them feel better.

But, even though everyday stress doesn't seem so harmful, it can do a lot of damage in the long run to both your weight and physiology. Interestingly enough, in the same study, 71 percent of the people who said they increased their consumption of unhealthy foods when stressed identify as "dieters," meaning they try to restrict these foods the rest of the time.

Unfortunately, this behavior doesn't just have an effect on your weight and the diseases associated with obesity (diabetes, heart disease, high blood pressure, etc.). Consistently self-medicating with carbohydrate-rich foods, for example, can lead to adaptations in our reward pathways and brain processes that will then make us depressed or anxious when these foods aren't available. Again, this is a behavior and adaptation similar to what we see in drug addiction.

So although highly palatable, often carbohydrate-rich comfort food can have an immediate positive effect on our well-being, it would be much more beneficial in the long term to have a variety of techniques you can use to help relieve stress or boost your spirits. Relying heavily on food to improve your mood will only backfire over time. Next time you're feeling down or anxious, look for other forms of support. Call a friend or family member, take a brisk walk, or sit down and read a few pages of a good book. Finding an activity that is exciting or interesting to you, that doesn't involve food or any potential food cues (such as streaming TV), will help you fulfill yourself emotionally in other ways without risking your health.

Food as a Drug

I mentioned before that some of the eating behaviors that we find ourselves engaged in often are similar to what we see with drug addiction. And it turns out that this isn't just a similarity. One of the reasons why sticking to a healthy eating plan can be so difficult has to do with the effect that the foods we eat can have on our brain and behavior. Due to the nature of the "obesity epidemic" in the United States, researchers have been scrambling to find a solution or cause for years. A significant amount of research (a lot of which has come out of my lab) has shown that eating a lot of highly processed foods that are rich in added sugars (like ice cream, cookies, and even pizza) can, over time, lead to changes in the brain that are like what happens when one becomes *addicted* to drugs or alcohol. This is part of the reason why it can be difficult to stick to a healthy diet: we are hooked on the junk food.

How exactly can we become addicted to junk food, and what can this mean for our health?

Although the addictiveness of junk food has not yet been extensively studied in humans (mostly because it's difficult to do so—have you ever met anyone who hasn't been eating junk food that could be in the control group? Probably not!), evidence from studies using laboratory animals supports the hypothesis that highly processed foods, especially those high in added sugar, may in fact be addictive. We also see that because of this, addictive eating behaviors develop in a very similar way to a drug or alcohol addiction.

When you eat highly processed foods that are typically high in fat and/or sugar, dopamine is released in the brain, creating the ultimate reward signal. When high amounts of dopamine are released, it makes us feel good about what we just ate, and usually our brain tells us we want more. The same is true if you come across a cue associated with food, such as the smell of cookies or popcorn. This will also elicit a dopamine response and increase your desire to have that food. Basically, this results in what we call "reward-driven" or "hedonic" eating. We are eating because it makes us feel good, not for the calories or nutrients.

From an evolutionary standpoint, this is an advantageous system.

Back when we were hunters and gatherers, finding palatable food in an environment where food was scarce allowed us to recognize that we should eat a lot of the food because it was unclear when the next meal would be. These days, however, food is anything but scarce, and our food environment is instead oversaturated with products containing excessive amounts of sugar. Although there are a variety of factors that contribute to weight gain, neuroimaging studies show that the dopamine reward system is altered in obese individuals in a way that is similar to individuals who are addicted to drugs of abuse.

From a fertility standpoint, a food addiction can be detrimental because not only is maintaining a healthy weight key to optimizing fertility, but also eating too much junk food (especially sugary foods) negatively impacts fertility. As you have probably begun to notice, a common theme throughout this book is the importance of eating mostly fresh, whole foods to increase your chances of having a baby.

• •

How Do I Know If I'm Addicted to Food?

- *You never feel satisfied when you eat healthy food.* You might feel more satisfied with junk food because of the immediate impact it has on the reward system in your brain. Healthier foods don't hijack the brain in the way that junk foods can to produce this effect.

- *You feel like you need to keep eating and eating to feel satisfied.* In animal and human studies, we see that overeating is common. In humans, however, it's not just because the food is rewarding—we feel that we need an increasing amount of food to feel satiated and satisfied. Our brains and bodies have an intricate system of signals in place to lead us to eat more, especially if the foods we are consuming don't contain all of the nutrients that we need to function at our best.

- *You are irritable and grumpy when dieting.* There is a plethora of research in animals that show how decreasing access to sugar causes an increase in anxiety, and we can often see the same in humans (you've probably even experienced this yourself at some point if you have cut back dramatically on sugar). Interestingly enough, one study was able to show that giving a carbohydrate-rich drink to women who were craving carbohydrates improved their mood.

- *You constantly crave certain foods.* Similar to being anxious or grumpy when dieting, research on food restriction shows us that when we restrict what we eat, we typically crave highly palatable foods such as candy, chips, fried foods, etc. Even more, when we finally have access to those foods again, we are more likely to overdo it and eat more than we should. You may have experienced something similar to this if you've ever been on a diet that restricts certain foods or food groups.

- *You engage in binge eating.* Binge eating is often considered a hallmark of food addiction. It involves rapidly consuming unusually large amounts of food in a short period of time. This behavior has been extensively studied in rats to show that an addicted individual may binge on food the way he or she may binge on drugs like alcohol.

Breaking the Association

Fortunately, humans are smart creatures and we have the capacity to change our goals, habits, and routines when we see fit. Breaking bad habits isn't impossible, but it can be difficult (thanks to dopamine). One obstacle we face is that breaking a bad habit such as eating sweets whenever you're tired means we have to replace an immediately rewarding habit with something that may be more rewarding in the long run, such as eating a fruit or nothing at all.

The good news is you don't have to try and change your habits all in one go. The best place to start is by simply trying to recognize and understand your habits. What are the triggers to your habits, and why do you engage in these behaviors? Once you are more conscious of your actions, you can come up with a plan to tackle them. One way to do this is by disrupting your habit—create your own obstacle that keeps you from engaging in this habit in the way that you normally would. For example, if you always hit snooze on your alarm clock before getting up, put your alarm away from your bed so that hitting snooze means you have to physically get out of bed and walk across the room. You can do the same thing when it comes to eating something that might not be healthy. If you are dying for a huge slice of pizza for dinner, go for it, but make the pizza yourself at home. When you do this, you will not only make it healthier than from a take-out place, but you will also put the effort in to prepare your own food, which will help you enjoy it even more.

One of the biggest mistakes people make when they decide to change their eating habits is to change too much too fast. Going "cold turkey" and trying to enact every change at the same time can leave you feeling exhausted, overwhelmed, and with no margin for error or slipup.

For the best results, you'll want to take baby steps and "wean off" of the foods that are doing you more harm than good. Cutting out certain foods altogether might make you more likely to indulge in unhealthy eating habits, such as bingeing.

Even though you don't have to start by completely replacing your habits all at once, you will want to do this sooner rather than later. Research shows that engaging in a replacement behavior, such as going for a walk when you're tired instead of reaching for sweets, increases the likelihood that you'll be able to break your old habits. At one point or another, finding something that you can do instead is key to erasing the habit and forming new ones. In doing so, you should also try to keep it simple. Choose something that is easy to implement and something that you can do habitually without too much effort.

Lastly, you'll have to be persistent and repetitive. Just as habits are formed through repetition, we won't be able to break them unless we consistently avoid them or engage in the replacement behavior. When you're feeling stuck, try to remind yourself of the long-term consequences or goal as an extra motivator. Even better, if you can find a replacement behavior with an immediate reward (i.e., an afternoon walk is more likely to make you less tired than loading up on sweets), you'll eventually look forward to getting the reward from this new habit when it comes time to engage in that behavior.

• •

Change Your Eating Habits for the Better

1. Find out what is triggering your cravings. Typically our cravings are related to some sort of cue, like an afternoon slump, or always having a pastry with your morning coffee. Does seeing candy on desks at the office make you crave sweets? Do you snack on chips when you're at home watching TV? Once you learn to recognize these triggers, you're one step further to making better decisions. Recognizing what tends to lead to cravings will allow you to stop and ask yourself, "Do I really need this?" or, "Am I really hungry right now?"

2. Since you're not quitting cold turkey, you'll need to manage your portion sizes when you do indulge. If you don't already portion out your food, you'll want to start now, especially when it comes to junk food. Instead of automatically limiting yourself to one serving size, think about how much you're currently eating, and then try to decrease the amount from there. Again, take baby steps. A good trick is to portion out your treats ahead of time by separating them into small containers or snack bags.

3. Are you the kind of person who eats things just because they're around you? Do you see something and automatically want to eat it? If so, "out of sight, out of mind" may be a good motto to have. Instead of leaving treats around the house or out in the open, put things away in drawers or in the refrigerator. Often we don't have cravings for a treat until we physically see it (or smell it), so if it's put away you won't be as tempted to reach for it. Better yet, don't bring junk food into your

house at all. Instead, if there's something you really want, you'll have to make an extra trip to the grocery store and go out of your way to get it.

4. While you're busy putting away your indulgent treats, make your healthy snacks as available as possible. Junk food is typically easily accessible, even if it's hidden away, which can often lead us to snacking on unhealthy things even if we're not necessarily craving it. Having healthy snacks like fruits, cut up veggies, plain yogurt, and dips like hummus or guacamole or healthy other options front and center in your refrigerator or on the counter at all times is key to making better choices.

• •

Dealing with Food Cravings

Do you ever have food cravings? If the answer to this question isn't "yes," I would be surprised. In fact, research tells us that food cravings are extremely common; in one study almost 100 percent of women and 70 percent of men reported having food cravings in the past year. With the overwhelming amount of highly palatable, "addicting" foods available in today's food environment, these numbers aren't surprising.

Considering the relationships among habits, mood, and tendency to self-medicate with food, it's no wonder that so many people experience food cravings at one point or another. Food cravings are defined as an intense desire to consume a particular food.

There's no one surefire way to deal with food cravings, but there are a variety of ways in which you can learn to manage them or decrease them.

1. *Get a good night's sleep.* Not getting enough sleep leads to several short- and long-term problems, especially when it comes to our food choices. In general, we see that insufficient sleep is associated with weight gain and overall increased food intake. More specifically, food cravings tend

to increase when you're sleepy, and we often gravitate toward high-fat and/or high-sugar foods. So not only are we eating more when we're tired, but we're eating more of the things we want to limit.

2. *Opt for whole foods over processed foods.* Considering what we know about the addictive qualities of highly palatable foods (especially those with a high sugar content), eating more whole foods and fewer processed foods is key to reducing food cravings. In addition, research shows us that eating a diet loaded with highly processed foods leads to weight gain, which is likely due in part to an increase in cravings.

3. *Practice portion control.* Even though we see that restriction of a certain food item can lead to increased cravings for that food, studies show that calorie restriction in general reduces overall food cravings. Thus, practicing portion control may be a helpful tool to help combat cravings if you have weight to lose.

4. *Reduce your everyday stress.* We touched upon this earlier, but it is important enough to talk about again. Stress in life can cause all sorts of problems. Eating can be a natural response to stress as a means to self-medicate, but stress can also induce food cravings. In some cases, stress is a trigger for cravings of highly palatable foods such as those with excessive sugar or fat (like candy or chips). As mentioned earlier, "routine" stress from our everyday lives may be small, but it's typically the most influential on our lives because it is so persistent. Finding ways to reduce everyday stressors will help minimize those stress-related cravings.

5. *Find a replacement food to satisfy your cravings.* Finding yummy alternatives to your favorite snacks or go-to items when a craving sets in will be a huge help in decreasing your intake of not-so-healthy foods. For example, eat 1–2 ounces of dark chocolate (70 percent or darker) when a chocolate craving sets in, eat frozen grapes instead of hard candies, try apples with raisins and cinnamon instead of

cookies, or drink peppermint tea instead of eating mint candies or cookies.

• •

Am I Really Hungry?

This is the million-dollar question. Cravings are a natural thing, and sometimes they are our body's way of letting us know that we need to eat something. However, cravings can also be triggered by stress, anxiety, or even our modern food environments (ever suddenly felt like getting a Frappuccino when you walked past Starbucks? That's the advertisement triggering a craving). So, it is important to ask yourself if you are actually hungry (i.e., is this a biologically driven craving for food because I am hungry?), or if you are seeking out the food for some other reason. Typically, when hunger-driven cravings occur, they are not for specific items (like ice cream), but rather for food groups (i.e., meats or pasta/carbs). So if you are getting a craving for peanut M&M's, you might need to put on the brakes and think about *why* you want it before you give in.

• •

◆ ◆ ◆

Hopefully this chapter helped you to do some self-reflecting and think about your habits (both good and bad), and how you can modify them to be healthier. Next, we are going to get into the specifics on which foods you can start to incorporate into your diet to boost your fertility.

CHAPTER 5

Twenty Foods You Should Eat to Boost Your Fertility

So far, we have covered a lot. We have reviewed the reasons why it is never too early to start thinking about improving your fertility with nutritional changes, and how what we eat can have a significant impact on our hormones and health. We have also reviewed which nutrients are important for fertility, why they are important, and which foods are rich in these nutrients. We have also covered some of the psychological aspects of eating well and how to navigate some of the barriers that come up when one tries to make changes in their diet, including managing cravings and changing unhealthy habits.

Now, it is time to get down to the details. In this chapter, I will lay out the twenty foods that you should try to incorporate into your diet to help boost your fertility. These foods were hand-picked because they are rich in one or more of the fertility-promoting nutrients that we discussed back in chapter 3. I'll go over why these foods are good for you and/or your partner, and also offer some recipe ideas that include them as primary ingredients. In chapter 7, I will provide some sample menus based on these recipes and other food ideas to help you plan out your meals and make it easier to eat healthy, nutritious foods while you are busy with other things (like getting pregnant).

As you go through this list, I suggest you pick out a few foods to focus on each week. That way, one week you can experiment yourself with creative ways to incorporate specific foods into your diet, and then next week change it up by trying a few more. There is really no right or wrong way to do this, and the plan is designed to be flexible and allow you to come up with fertility-boosting food swaps to make in your own diet.

Fertility-Boosting Food: Wheat Bran

Wheat bran is not only an excellent source of magnesium, but it also provides a little more than half of the selenium that you need for the day. It's crazy that bran is often viewed as just a "by-product" when grains are milled, when in reality it is a nutrient powerhouse! It's a great source of omega-3 fatty acids, and it is loaded with anti-oxidants. Because inflammation has been shown to negatively impact pregnancy, boosting your antioxidant intake is a great way to combat damaging free radicals. Plus, because low levels of omega-3 fatty acids have been associated with decreased ability to get pregnant, it is a great idea to incorporate more foods rich in omega-3s into your diet. Wheat bran also contains lignans, and these provide us with phytoestrogens. Phytoestrogens behave similarly to estrogens in our body. It is thought that lignans may help increase endometrial thickness, which is beneficial for the embryo.

• •

Aren't Phytoestrogens Bad for Fertility?

Phytoestrogens are plant-derived compounds found in foods such as soy products, grains, beans, and some fruits and vegetables. Some reports claim that since phytoestrogens can mimic estrogens, they may act as "endocrine disruptors." It turns out that although they can mimic the effects that natural estrogens have in the body, that isn't always a bad thing. In fact, there is actually a lot of research that explores the health benefits of phytoestrogens, including their ability to help reduce total cholesterol and improve heart function, and even the prevention of other chronic diseases, such as type 2 diabetes, cancer, and obesity. These findings seem to fall in line with the health benefits seen by those eating a plant-based diet, which is also a diet rich in phytoestrogens. When it comes to female fertility, phytoestrogens may be helpful. In a study examining the outcomes of women undergoing infertility treatment, the odds of achieving a successful live birth were higher for women in the group that had the highest intake of phytoestrogen-packed dietary soy. On the other hand, when it comes to *male* fertility, the effect of phytoestrogens does not seem to be as positive. Recent research is uncovering that perhaps there is a relationship between phytoestrogen exposure and infertility, such that an increase in exposure to phytoestrogens (such as through eating more soy products) may lead to an increase in abnormal sperm, lower sperm counts, and decreased sperm motility.

So, should men avoid phytoestrogens? Not completely. Men definitely should *not* stop eating a plant-based diet or eat fewer vegetables. Instead, if men want to reduce intake of phytoestrogens, they might consider cutting down on soy intake (tofu, tempeh, edamame, soy sauce, etc.), and be sure to read the ingredients list on any supplements, as soy might be included.

• •

Now's the time to start incorporating wheat bran into your diet. The good news is that wheat bran isn't a fancy "health food" that is going to cost a fortune. It's easy to find in the supermarket, and adding ½ cup to some of your favorite recipes is an easy way to start eating more of it. Try the Overnight Protein-Powered Oats with Berries or a fresh batch of the Banana-Bran Pancakes to get some wheat bran into your diet, and enjoy!

Overnight Protein-Powered Oats with Berries

If you are looking for a healthy and easy way to start your day, look no further. Overnight oats are easy to prepare the night before, and the protein will help you to start off your day feeling great. Plus, the wheat bran and fruit in these will give you a boost of antioxidants and phytoestrogens.

Makes 1 serving.

½ cup	rolled oats
½ cup	milk of your choice: almond coconut, dairy, etc.
1 tablespoon	wheat bran
1 teaspoon	maple syrup
pinch	sea salt
	choice of mixed berries: raspberry, blueberry, strawberry, or strawberry, banana, or pineapple
1 tablespoon	slivered almonds or crushed walnuts (optional)

Add oats, milk, wheat bran, maple syrup, and salt into 8-ounce container. Stir to combine. Add toppings of your choice. Cover tightly with plastic wrap or mason jar lid and refrigerate overnight. In the morning, mix in nuts (optional) and eat cold straight from jar or add a little milk and rewarm in the microwave.

Banana-Bran Pancakes

Pancakes are great for any meal, and the leftovers make for a nutritious snack. These pancakes have banana bits instead of mashed bananas, so you get the added texture and taste. Sifting might seem like a chore, but it will help to ensure that the pancakes are fluffy.

Makes about 10 pancakes.

1½ cups	milk
1 cup	oats
¾ cup	sifted all-purpose flour
¼ cup	wheat bran
1 tablespoon	baking powder
1 teaspoon	salt
2	eggs, beaten
¼ cup	melted butter or margarine
1	medium banana, cut into bite-size pieces

In a mixing bowl, pour the milk over the oats and let them stand for 5 minutes. Add the flour, wheat bran, baking powder, and salt. Mix in the eggs and butter, stirring with a spoon until combined. Ladle in batches on to a greased or nonstick griddle or frying pan over medium heat. Add pieces of banana on top of the pancake, and cook until the tops are bubbly and the edges look cooked. Turn over and finish cooking the other side.

• •

Healthful Tip

Make sure to store your wheat bran in an airtight container, and keep it in the refrigerator or freezer to prevent it from going rancid. Sealing it up correctly will allow it to last for up to a year (but hopefully you'll love it so much, it won't last that long).

• •

Fertility-Boosting Food: Avocado

Luckily, avocados have become very popular, so you may already be eating them regularly. Go out to any restaurant for brunch, and avocado toast will likely be on the menu, and for a good reason: Avocados are delicious!

Unlike other fruits, avocados are calorically dense. Just 1/5 of this fruit yields about 50 calories due to the fat content. Not to worry though, as the majority of fat from avocados are heart-healthy monounsaturated fatty acids (MUFAs). Researchers have found that when women replaced trans fats with MUFAs, the risk of infertility related to ovulation function and inflammation significantly decreased. Like all fruits, avocados do have carbohydrates, but they also have significantly more fiber. For example, when compared to a banana weighing the same amount, there is less than half the carbohydrate and almost triple the fiber, making avocado's glycemic index almost nonexistent. Additionally, avocados are high in potassium, vitamin C, and magnesium, which all positively impact fertility.

Are All Fats the Same?

Fat has a bad rap as being unhealthy for your diet, but that isn't entirely true. Some fats are unhealthy, while others are an important part of a healthy diet. Here is a quick breakdown of the different types of fats that we commonly find in foods:

- *Monounsaturated fatty-acids (MUFAs):* These fats are considered healthy fats. They can help reduce "bad" cholesterol and lower your risk for heart disease.

- *Saturated fats:* You want to avoid these fats. They can increase your cholesterol and risk for heart disease and stroke.

- *Trans fats:* These are also the fats we want to avoid. Studies show that they can increase triglyceride and cholesterol levels, and they can also increase risk for heart disease.

- *Omega-3 fatty acids:* These are considered healthy fats, but they can be high in calories, so eat foods that contain them in moderation.

If you haven't already been smearing avocado on your bread or chopping it up into a salad, what are you waiting for? Try the Egg and Avocado Breakfast Sandwich or just make yourself a nice bowl of Avocado "Pesto" and Pasta. The Buffalo Cauliflower "Wings" with Avocado Aioli Dipping Sauce (page 84) is also a great option for a side or late-night healthy snack, and the Fertility-Friendly "Sushi" Bowl (page 70) makes for a quick and healthy lunch or dinner.

Egg and Avocado Breakfast Sandwich

Poached eggs are not only yummy, but they are healthier than their fried or scrambled counterparts because you don't need to use oil or butter to prepare them. The avocado gives this sandwich a smooth taste, and also some fertility-friendly potassium, vitamin C and magnesium.

Makes 1 sandwich.

2 slices	whole-grain bread
½	avocado, sliced
1 teaspoon	white vinegar (to poach the egg)
½ teaspoon	salt
1	egg
pinch	cayenne
	salt and pepper to taste

Toast the bread and place slices of avocado on one piece. Fill a saucepan with water and place over medium heat. Add salt and vinegar and bring to a gentle simmer, then reduce heat to low. Crack the egg into a ramekin, and then gently pour it into the water. Cook for about 6 minutes, then use a slotted spoon to remove it. Place egg on top of avocado. Add cayenne, salt, and pepper. Top the sandwich with the other slice of toasted bread.

Avocado "Pesto" and Pasta

This healthier take on traditional pesto sauce uses antioxidant-rich cilantro instead of basil, giving you an extra kick of vitamin K, folate, and potassium. The addition of the avocado gives not only added nutrients and healthy fats, but also gives a smooth taste that pairs well with the cheese.

Makes 6 servings.

12 ounces	dry pasta (elbows or cavatappi work well)
2	avocados, peeled and pitted
¼ cup	fresh cilantro
2 tablespoons	lime juice
3 tablespoons	butter
3 tablespoons	flour
1½ cups	milk
1½ cups	shredded white cheddar cheese

Cook the pasta according to the package directions, until it is al dente. In a food processor, combine the avocado, cilantro, and lime juice and pulse until a creamy sauce forms. In a saucepan, melt butter over medium heat. Whisk in the flour, and cook for about a minute, whisking constantly. Slowly whisk in the milk, and cook until the sauce thickens, for about 5 minutes, again whisking constantly. Whisk in the avocado mixture and cook for another 2 minutes. Remove from heat, and mix in the cheddar cheese until it has melted. Add pasta, and toss until pasta is coated.

• •

Storage Tip

Add some lemon or lime juice to the exposed avocado fruit to prevent it from browning (the acid will help prevent oxidation) and store it in an airtight container. Avocados don't last long, so plan to use any leftovers in the next day.

• •

Fertility-Boosting Food: Whole-Grain Bread

If you're someone who typically chooses "white" over "whole-grain" breads, it's time to start making the healthier swap. For some people it is difficult, especially if you've been eating the white variety your entire life, so if this is you, start to slowly incorporate it. There are a plethora of health reasons why making the change is beneficial, especially when it comes to fertility. Not only do whole grains provide fiber, antioxidants, and vitamins, they also contain minerals and "antinutrients" like phytic acid. Phytates are often called antinutrients because they can decrease the absorption of certain minerals, but recently the scientific community has started to change its mind on them. They are mainly found in grains, and not only are they associated with decreased prevalence of cardiovascular disease, but they also exhibit anti-inflammatory properties. As we have already noted, inflammation is an enemy of fertility. However, the positive link between intake of whole grains and fertility is not only due to the anti-inflammation effects but also related to improved glucose control and insulin levels. Moreover, one study found that women who consumed more whole grains prior to in vitro fertilization (IVF) treatment were more likely to have a live birth, which the authors speculate may be due to increased endometrial thickness on the day that they received the embryo. So hopefully you're convinced that it's worth retraining your taste buds to go for whole grain over white when it comes to bread, and I promise that eventually you may even prefer it!

Whole grains provide a denser texture and a hearty flavor. Try out the Egg and Avocado Breakfast Sandwich (page 66), which is prepared using whole-grain bread, or this Macadamia-Nut "Ricotta" Toast with Honey Glaze.

Macadamia-Nut "Ricotta" Toast with Honey Glaze

Move over, avocado toast. Faux ricotta is now a thing, and it is about to become your new favorite toast topping. The macadamia nuts give this dish flavor, as well as many important fertility-friendly nutrients, including calcium. Using whole-grain bread instead of white bread makes this dish even healthier.

Makes 1 serving.

1 cup	raw macadamia nuts
1 teaspoon	salt
	juice from ½ medium lemon
¼ cup	water
1 slice	whole-grain bread
1 tablespoon	honey

In a food processor, combine macadamia nuts, salt, lemon juice, and water. Pulse until smooth, scraping down the sides as needed. Add additional water 1 tablespoon at a time if needed. Toast the bread. Spread the "ricotta" mixture on the toast. Drizzle with honey. You can store the leftover "ricotta" in the refrigerator for up to 3 days.

• •

Healthful Hint

"Multigrain" bread is NOT the same as "whole grain"—multigrain just means that there are several different kinds of grains in a particular type of bread. So if you do choose a multigrain variety instead of a single grain bread (e.g., wheat or rye) make sure that it says "WHOLE MULTIGRAIN," or you're likely just getting glorified white bread.

• •

Fertility-Boosting Food: Farro

Farro is a grain that has been around for thousands of years, but is not nearly as popular as other grains like rice or couscous. This is surprising, because it provides a delicious flavor, a chewy texture, and almost quadruple the amount of fiber compared to rice. Plus, only ½ cup of farro provides a whopping 7 grams of protein. Like other whole grains, farro is also a good source of key minerals including zinc. Being low on this micronutrient is never good, especially when trying to conceive. If you recall from chapter 3, zinc is needed for countless reactions within the body, including rapidly dividing cells and producing healthy eggs! In fact, suboptimal maternal zinc levels have been associated with complications throughout pregnancy as well as fetal loss. Additionally, zinc deficiency can contribute to iron deficiency anemia, so it's important that your diet has adequate amounts of it. The good news is that only ½ cup of cooked farro (about the size of a tennis ball) gives you 15 percent of your daily zinc needs. Just like other grains, make sure it says "whole" and avoid the "pearled" form, which has the outermost bran layer removed during processing, stripping it of key nutrients.

Farro can take 30–40 minutes to cook, so it is best to make a large batch. It tastes great sprinkled in cold salads, added to any hearty soup, or used as a breakfast grain (try it instead of oatmeal). Try the yummy Fertility-Friendly "Sushi" Bowl, which uses farro instead of rice for a heartier texture and a nutritional boost.

Fertility-Friendly "Sushi" Bowl

It can be a challenge for sushi lovers to enjoy it when trying to get pregnant because of fears of mercury and toxins in fish. This sushi bowl is not only safe for those who are trying to conceive but also packed with fertility-boosting nutrients like zinc, omega-3s, and calcium.

Makes 2 servings.

2 cups	cooked farro
4 ounces	smoked salmon, sliced
1	raw carrot, shredded
1	cucumber, sliced
1	avocado, peeled, pitted, and sliced
1 packet	nori seaweed snack, torn into smaller pieces
4 tablespoons	mayonnaise
2 tablespoons	sriracha
1 tablespoon	sesame seeds

Place cooked farro in the bottom of your serving bowl. Arrange salmon, carrot, cucumber, and avocado on top. Add a few pieces of seaweed snack. In a separate bowl, mix together mayonnaise and sriracha, then drizzle over sushi bowl. Top with sesame seeds.

Fertility-Boosting Food: Sweet Potatoes

Sweet potatoes are a delicious root vegetable packed with vitamins, minerals, and anti-inflammatory compounds. Sweet potatoes are good sources of vitamins A and C, potassium, and vitamins B_3 and B_6. If you recall from chapter 3, many of these vitamins are helpful for fertility. Whenever picking them out at the store, aim for the brightest or darkest in color—these will be the richest in antioxidants. Remember, the more colorful the skin, the better. Since flavors will also vary (based on the type and color) it's a good excuse to expand your palate by replacing the white potato with a sweet variety instead.

Sweet potatoes taste great simply baked in the oven or they also can be used for homemade fries or breakfast hash. Try the Lamb and Sweet Potato Pie for a hearty, healthy dish that will satisfy your hunger and is packed with fertility-boosting nutrition. Or, whip up Easy Turmeric Turkey, Sweet Potato, and Zucchini Bowl. For breakfast ideas, check out the Garlicky Spinach Omelet with Sweet Potato Mash on page 87.

Lamb and Sweet Potato Pie

Pie isn't just for dessert. The sweet potatoes in this dish give you a boost of fertility-friendly vitamin A, vitamin C, and vitamin B_6. The lamb is a leaner alternative to beef, and very flavorful.

Makes about 6 servings.

1½ pounds	ground lamb
2	celery sticks, chopped
2	carrots, peeled and sliced thin
½	medium onion, chopped
3	medium garlic cloves, minced
1 14-ounce can	crushed tomatoes
2 tablespoons	fresh oregano, chopped
1 teaspoon	cinnamon
2 teaspoons	ground cumin
1 tablespoon	olive oil
2	large sweet potatoes, peeled and sliced ⅛ inch thick

Preheat oven to 350° F. In a bowl, mix together ground lamb, celery, carrots, onion, garlic, and tomatoes. Add the oregano, cinnamon, and cumin. Make sure mixture is well combined. Pour olive oil into a Dutch oven, and place half of the sweet potato slices in a single layer on the bottom (overlapping as needed so there are no spaces). Place the lamb mixture on top. Add remaining sweet potatoes in a single layer on top. Bake in the oven uncovered for 1 hour, then cover and bake for another 30 minutes. Remove from heat and let rest for 30 minutes before serving.

Easy Turmeric Turkey, Sweet Potato, and Zucchini Bowl

This is a great recipe to help you get the nutrients you need to boost your fertility, yet also easy to prepare and great for meal prep. This recipe is rich in fertility-promoting iron, phosphorus, potassium, zinc, and vitamin A. Make a big batch and package separately so you can quickly heat it up and eat throughout the week.

Makes 4 servings.

2	sweet potatoes (medium, sliced into rounds)
3 tablespoons	extra-virgin olive oil, divided
2	zucchini (medium, sliced into rounds)
1 pound	extra-lean ground turkey
2 teaspoons	turmeric
1 teaspoon	cumin
½ teaspoon	sea salt
2 tablespoons	tahini

Preheat oven to 425° F. Toss the sweet potatoes in 1 tablespoon of the olive oil and spread out on a baking sheet. Bake for 15 minutes. Take the sweet potatoes out, flip them, and move to one side of the baking sheet. Toss the zucchini in 1 tablespoon of the olive oil and put on the other side of the baking sheet (or another one if no room). Put the zucchini and sweet potato back in the oven for another 15 minutes. In the meantime, heat the remaining tablespoon of olive oil in a skillet over medium heat. Add the ground turkey and brown. Once the turkey is cooked through, add turmeric, cumin, and sea salt and mix well. Turn off the heat, remove the sweet potato and zucchini from the oven, and divide the items among four plates. Drizzle tahini on top of each plate before serving.

Fertility-Boosting Food: Peppers

Whether you favor the green bell peppers or the red and orange varieties, peppers are a nutrient dense food that is refreshing when eaten cold and slightly sweet when roasted. Although red bell peppers do contain more vitamin C and beta-carotene compared to the green ones, all peppers are low in calories and a good source of fiber. Peppers are not only a lighter alternative to have in place of chips as a crunchy snack, but they are packed with phytochemicals, vitamins, and minerals to help support fertility. Beta-carotene, lutein, flavonoids, and lycopene are just a few compounds that are found in bell peppers and help reduce inflammation throughout the body and may play a role in ovulation as well.

Plus, when cooked alongside an iron-rich veggie or bean, the vitamin C from the pepper will improve your absorption of the non-heme iron. That is why I have paired sliced red peppers for dipping with the Homemade Lemon Hummus. If you need a dinner idea, try the Cherry-Glazed Chicken Kebabs (page 105), or the Roasted Pepper and Parmesan Cauliflower Florets as a side dish.

Homemade Lemon Hummus

Hummus is a Mediterranean diet staple, and it isn't that hard to make. Just toss these ingredients into the food processor, and you will have a healthy snack in a snap. Ditch the pita chips and enjoy with nutrient-packed pepper slices, instead.

1	(15-ounce) can garbanzo beans (also known as chickpeas), drained and rinsed
¼ cup	tahini
2 tablespoons	warm water
2 tablespoons	olive oil
6 tablespoons	lemon juice
1 tablespoon	ground cumin
½ teaspoon	salt

pepper (to taste)
1   red bell pepper, sliced

In a food processor, combine garbanzo beans, tahini, water, olive oil, lemon juice, cumin and salt. Pulse until smooth and creamy. Add to a serving bowl, and add pepper to taste. Serve alongside sliced peppers for dipping. Store leftover hummus in the refrigerator for up to 3 days.

Roasted Pepper and Parmesan Cauliflower Florets

Alone, cauliflower is amazing and full of fertility-promoting nutrients, like vitamin C and folate. This side dish pairs cauliflower with peppers to add flavor, different texture, and more nutrients.

Makes 4 servings.

1   whole cauliflower, cut into florets
2   red bell peppers, sliced
4 tablespoons   olive oil
½ cup   grated Parmesan cheese
salt and pepper to taste

Preheat oven to 400° F. Place cauliflower florets and pepper slices in a bowl and coat with olive oil. Add cheese. Add salt and pepper to taste. Spread onto a baking sheet, and roast for 30 minutes.

Fertility-Boosting Food: Brazil Nuts

Brazil nuts contain high amounts of selenium, which is essential for reproductive health. Besides being an excellent source of selenium (just 4–5 nuts provide the recommended amount of selenium needed per day, so don't eat them in excess because more than that amount can lead to selenium toxicity), these nuts are also high in MUFA and vitamin C. They are energy dense (about six provide almost 200 calories) and are good for both male and female reproduction. In fact, they have been shown to increase testosterone levels and sperm count. Getting pregnant may be your *main* goal right now, but keeping your heart healthy should be a high priority as well (especially since there is a relationship between heart disease and infertility). The good news is that Brazil nuts likely help improve your heart health due to their abundance of healthy fats. After eating just one serving, research shows that patients had actually improved HDL (good cholesterol) levels and lower LDL (bad cholesterol)!

So, next time you're going to throw some nuts in your salad, switch out the slivered almonds and chop up a couple of Brazil nuts instead. The Mixed Green Salad with Fertility-Boosting Nutty-Basil Vinaigrette is a great option for lunch or a side at dinner. Need a light dinner or late-night snack and looking for something new and exciting? Check out the Fertility-Friendly "Prosecco" with Nut and Cheese Tapas (page 156) for something more indulgent!

Mixed Green Salad with Fertility-Boosting Nutty-Basil Vinaigrette

This light side dish pairs well with pretty much any main course. The pairing of basil and Brazil nuts in the dressing gives this salad a unique flavor that also helps to boost your selenium intake.

Makes 2 servings.

½ cup	fresh basil leaves, packed
1 clove	garlic
4	Brazil nuts
½ cup	extra-virgin olive oil
2 tablespoons	lemon juice
¼ teaspoon	salt
¼ teaspoon	ground pepper
4 cups	mixed salad greens

In a food processor, combine basil, garlic, and Brazil nuts. Pulse until the nuts are coarsely chopped. Add in olive oil, lemon juice, salt, and pepper. Plate the mixed salad greens, and add dressing on top or serve on the side.

Fertility-Boosting Food: Sardines

Even though sardines are cheap and highly nutritious, they seem to be more popular in other countries than in the United States. So, if this is a fish you typically stay away from, now is the time to change that.

Besides Brazil nuts, seafood is another excellent source of selenium, with sardines being one of the best. This trace mineral not only acts as an antioxidant, thus protecting our cells from damage, but it is needed to keep glucose levels under control, which is vital when trying to get pregnant. Further, sardines are low in mercury and one of the few good food sources of vitamin D. If you're going for the canned variety, purchase sardines in olive oil, not soy oil. One study found that women who consumed a diet high in fish and olive oil prior to becoming pregnant actually had a higher likelihood of embryo growth. Just pop open a can and add them to the Mixed Green Salad with Fertility-Boosting Nutty-Basil Vinaigrette (page 76) for a meal with an additional source of healthy fats and protein. But if you need something fast, they also taste great on their own with some fresh-squeezed lemon and parsley. Feeling fancy? Mix in some capers for a briny kick. Try the Grilled Sardine and Cashew Shrimp Stir-Fry for a delicious dinner, and you can take any leftovers for lunch the next day.

Grilled Sardine and Cashew Shrimp Stir-Fry

This recipe has a blend of all the nutrients that specifically support male fertility, in addition to ample protein, healthy fat, and fiber. Shrimp and sardines provide selenium, while the cashews and peppers provide zinc and vitamin C (among many other essential nutrients). Not to mention, this recipe is super quick, delicious, and well-rounded to keep you satisfied.

Makes 4 servings.

1 pound	medium shrimp, peeled and deveined
2 tablespoons	sesame oil
1	red bell pepper, chopped
1 tablespoon	ginger, finely grated
2 cloves	garlic, finely chopped
	red pepper flakes to taste
1–2 tablespoons	soy sauce
½	lime
½ cup	roasted cashews, chopped
1	(4-ounce) can sardines
	steamed brown rice (or farro) for serving

Pat the shrimp dry with a paper towel. Heat a large skillet over high heat with sesame oil. Carefully add the shrimp in a single layer and let cook for 1 minute. Continue to cook for 1 to 2 minutes more, stirring occasionally, until almost cooked through. Add the pepper, ginger, garlic, and red pepper flakes if desired, cooking for 1 more minute. Add the soy sauce and the juice from half a lime, cooking for 1 more minute. When finished, stir in cashews and sardines and serve over rice or farro.

Fertility-Boosting Food: Tomatoes

This one is especially for the guys! As we have discussed throughout, boosting men's fertility is just as important as boosting women's. Did you know that foods rich in lycopene, such as tomatoes, can help improve sperm motility and health? Studies conducted on both humans and animals have shown promising results in lycopene alleviating male infertility: sperm count and viability were increased. Human trials have reported improvement in sperm parameters and pregnancy rates with supplementation of 4–8 mg of lycopene daily for 3–12 months. But here is the really important point: Lycopene is highest in *processed* tomatoes, so instead of opting for tomatoes in your salad, order the pasta sauce instead!

To get more lycopene in your diet, try the Vegetarian "Meatballs" with Tomato Sauce, or the Eggplant and Orzo with Turmeric and Tomato Sauce. Meat eater? Check out the Lamb and Sweet Potato Pie on page 72 (there are tomatoes in it!)

Vegetarian "Meatballs" with Tomato Sauce

There are many health benefits of eating a plant-based diet, and now you can enjoy your favorite meat dishes without the guilt. This vegetarian version of meatballs pairs great with pasta, and the tomato sauce gives you a health boost of fertility-friendly lycopene.

Makes about 15 small meatballs.

3 tablespoons	olive oil
1	medium onion, chopped
20 ounces	portobello mushrooms, finely chopped
4 cloves	garlic, minced
1 cup	quick-cooking oats
1 cup	bread crumbs
½ cup	parsley, chopped
2	eggs
½ teaspoon	dried oregano
1	(24-ounce) jar marinara sauce

Preheat oven to 400° F. Add oil to a skillet over medium heat and sauté the onion for about 5 minutes. Add mushrooms and cook for 10 minutes or until they brown. Add garlic and remove from heat.

Once the mushroom mixture has cooled, add it to a bowl and combine with oats, bread crumbs, parsley, eggs, and oregano. Stir the mixture well and cover it with cellophane and refrigerate overnight. When ready to cook, make small balls (a little larger than a golf ball) and bake them for 15 minutes. Add marinara sauce to a medium saucepan. Once the meatballs are done in the oven, add them to the marinara sauce and cook over low heat for 15 minutes.

Eggplant and Orzo with Turmeric and Tomato Sauce

This vegan dish is not only filling, but also loaded with nutrients like lycopene from the tomato sauce and iron from the orzo and turmeric. You don't need to peel the eggplant before you cook it. The outer part is completely edible and softens when you roast it.

Makes 4 servings.

3	medium eggplant (about 2 pounds total), cut into ½-inch-thick rounds
3 tablespoons	olive oil
	salt and pepper, to taste
4 cups	cooked orzo, warm or at room temperature
1	(24-ounce) jar marinara sauce
1	(15-ounce) can garbanzo beans, drained and rinsed
¼ cup	coarsely chopped fresh mint leaves
½ teaspoon	turmeric

Preheat oven to 400° F. Place the eggplant in a single layer on a baking sheet and drizzle with olive oil and salt and pepper. Roast for 15 minutes, then flip the slices and roast for 10 minutes more.

Divide the orzo among four bowls and add marinara sauce on top. Top with the eggplant and garbanzo beans. Sprinkle with the mint and turmeric.

Fertility-Boosting Food: Pomegranate

Who doesn't love a juicy tart pomegranate? Yes, they can be annoying to open, especially since they stain pretty much everything, but thankfully the Internet is chock full of videos showing you how to "easily" open a pomegranate. Pomegranates are loaded with different flavonoids that have been implicated in an array of health benefits. Some of the more popular compounds include quercetin and anthocyanins. Not only has quercetin been shown to play a role in keeping our immune system strong, but it also exhibits anti-inflammatory properties, which has a beneficial effect on fertility.

Anthocyanins are another class of compounds that are also found in other fruits and vegetables (responsible for giving specific foods their blue, red, and purple hues) and are also anti-inflammatory. Plus, research shows that these compounds help offset the negative impact that exposure to environmental pollutants has on fertility.

Pomegranate tastes great on its own as a simple snack, but is also delicious when incorporated into a Middle Eastern–inspired lamb dish (try some on top of the Lamb and Sweet Potato Pie, page 72). If you're not one for sweet and savory in the same dish, opt to make your breakfast a little more anti-inflammatory by topping the Waffles with Honey-Sweetened Frozen Yogurt (page 155) with ½ cup of pomegranate seeds. Be sure to try the Cashew and Pomegranate Granola Cereal or the Savory Mushroom, Onion and Thyme Oats.

• •

Healthy Hint:

Since pomegranates aren't necessarily the cheapest of the fruits to purchase, you want to make sure you pick a winner. Choose one that feels "heavy" for its size, and stay away from ones that have areas of soft spots.

• •

Cashew and Pomegranate Granola Cereal

Making your own granola is a great way to make sure it includes all of your favorite ingredients, like fertility-boosting pomegranate and yummy nuts and seeds. You can use this granola as a snack, breakfast cereal, or topping for yogurt. It stores in an airtight container for about a month, so this recipe is for a large batch.

Makes about 10 servings.

2½ cups	old-fashioned oats
1 cup	cooked quinoa
1 cup	sliced almonds
1 cup	cashews, chopped
1 cup	roasted and salted sunflower seeds
⅓ cup	toasted sesame seeds
1 cup	pomegranate seeds
¾ cup	pure maple syrup
¼ cup	coconut oil
1 teaspoon	vanilla extract
1 teaspoon	nutmeg
1 teaspoon	cinnamon
1 teaspoon	salt

Preheat oven to 325° F. In a large bowl, mix together the oats, quinoa, almonds, cashews, sunflower seeds, sesame seeds, and pomegranate seeds. In a small saucepan, heat the maple syrup, coconut oil, vanilla, nutmeg, cinnamon, and salt over medium heat for 2–3 minutes until blended. Pour the mixture over the oats and toss for a couple of minutes to make sure everything is fully combined. Spread the granola out in an even layer on baking sheet lined with parchment, and press down with a spatula to flatten it. Bake for 45–50 minutes, stirring 2–3 times. Remove the granola from the oven and let sit for 5 minutes. Once slightly cooled, use a spatula to flatten it again and let cool for at least an hour before serving.

Savory Mushroom, Onion, and Thyme Oats

This dish is versatile (good for breakfast, lunch, or dinner), and full of so many fertility promoting nutrients. Altogether, you'll find plenty of fiber, iron, B vitamins, magnesium, calcium, vitamin D (especially if you use portobello mushrooms), and potassium in this dish, along with the benefits of pomegranate. We often think of oatmeal as a sweet or bland breakfast dish, but hopefully this recipe will show you that we can get the fiber from oatmeal without sacrificing taste. For a shorter cooking time, use rolled oats in place of steel-cut oats, and add a boiled egg on top for a protein and calorie boost.

Makes about 2 to 4 servings.

2 cups	water (or 1 cup for rolled oats)
1 cup	steel-cut oats
2 tablespoons	olive oil
½	medium onion, finely sliced
2 cloves	garlic, minced
6–8 ounces	any edible mushroom (cremini, shiitake, portobello, baby bella)
3–5 sprigs	thyme, leaves removed, discard stems
⅓ cup	pomegranate seeds
⅓ cup	chopped walnuts
	sea salt and pepper to taste

Bring water to boil in a medium size pot. Add oats, and cover. Let simmer for 25 to 30 minutes (for rolled oats, cooking time is reduced to about 5 to 8 minutes, depending on how mushy you like the texture). Heat the oil in a saucepan over medium heat, then add the onion and garlic. Sauté for about 3 minutes, then add mushrooms and thyme, cooking until the mushrooms are golden brown. To serve, put the oatmeal in the pan to mix everything together, place in a bowl, and top with pomegranate, chopped walnuts, salt, and pepper.

Fertility-Boosting Food: Cauliflower

Cauliflower has definitely increased in popularity lately, and rightfully so! This cruciferous vegetable is often subbed in as a lower-carb option for mashed potatoes, rice or pizza crust. It's a good thing that not only is it versatile and tasty, but it's exceptionally high in many key nutrients associated with pregnancy. One cup of cauliflower contains only about 25 calories but delivers almost 80 percent of your daily vitamin C, 20 percent of your vitamin K, and 15 percent of your daily folate needs. Plus it's a good source of fiber, and cruciferous veggies are associated with deceased risk of cardiovascular disease and blood clots. We know that high blood sugar levels are associated with negative pregnancy outcomes, and cauliflower may even help with that! One study found that phytochemicals in cauliflower actually inhibited the enzymes that break down starchy carbohydrates, which would aid in improved blood sugar control.

Cauliflower can also be used as a substitute for chips when you're craving your favorite creamy dips. If you're trying to cut back on meat, try the Buffalo Cauliflower "Wings" with Avocado Aioli Dipping Sauce, which are always a crowd pleaser, or you can also try replacing the potatoes with mashed cauliflower in the Lamb and Sweet Potato Pie (page 72). Or, try the Roasted Pepper and Parmesan Cauliflower Florets (page 75)

Buffalo Cauliflower "Wings" with Avocado Aioli Dipping Sauce

This is a lower-calorie meat-free version of Buffalo chicken wings, so you can enjoy them without the guilt. Make them for your next half-time party, and you will see that they are a hit! If you want to make this dish vegan, use oat milk instead of cow's milk, and swap out the butter for 2 tablespoons of olive oil, instead.

Makes 4 servings.

FOR THE "WINGS"

½	large head cauliflower, cut into florets
4 tablespoons	olive oil
¼ cup	almond meal
¼ teaspoon	garlic powder
2 tablespoons	milk
½ cup	Buffalo sauce or hot sauce
4 teaspoons	melted butter

FOR THE AIOLI

1	avocado, pitted and peeled
3 cloves	garlic
1 teaspoon	dried parsley
2 tablespoons	lemon juice
2 tablespoons	white wine vinegar
	salt to taste
½ cup	avocado oil
¼ cup	extra-virgin olive oil

Preheat oven to 425° F. Add cauliflower florets to a bowl and coat with olive oil. Add almond meal and garlic powder, and continue to mix. Add milk. Arrange in a single layer on a baking sheet lined with parchment paper, and bake for 25 minutes. In a separate bowl, combine the Buffalo sauce and melted butter. When the cauliflower florets are done cooking, remove them from the oven and once cool, dip them into the sauce. Bake for another 15 minutes.

For the avocado aioli, combine the avocado, garlic, parsley, lemon juice, vinegar, and salt and puree until smooth, scraping down the sides. With the machine running, add the oils and blend until emulsified. Serve alongside the baked cauliflower florets.

• •

Healthful Hint:

If you happen to see the purple variety of cauliflower, give it a shot. The richer color is prettier than the white variety, and this color means that it has more phytonutrients, including anthocyanins, flavonoids, resveratrol, and phenolic acids. All these polyphenols work hard to decrease inflammation, which is helpful for a successful pregnancy!

• •

Fertility-Boosting Food: Spinach

Spinach is replete with nutrients needed to support a healthy baby: fiber, choline, folate, iron, magnesium, and vitamin A just to name a few. Since folate protects against neural tube defects and is needed during any period of rapid growth and cell division, all women of childbearing potential should make sure they are getting enough. In addition to these key nutrients, spinach is also an excellent source of nitrates. Nitrates are a special kind of phytochemical that are beneficial for heart health because they reduce blood pressure and increase blood flow within tissues. Additionally, spinach may also improve exercise tolerance by regulating the usage of oxygen in our muscles, which is good news, because physical activity is associated with better chances of becoming pregnant!

. . . .

Aren't Nitrates Bad for You?

If you are keeping up with the do's and don'ts of what to eat when you do become pregnant, you probably have read that you should avoid foods that contain nitrates (like in bacon or deli meats). This is because some suggest that nitrates that are often added to meats to cure and preserve them have been linked to cancer. However, spinach (and many other vegetables) contains nitrates, so should you avoid it, too? No way! The reason is that the nitrates found in food (even bacon) aren't usually a problem until they are exposed to very high heat, when they can create nitrosamines—these are carcinogens. When you cook bacon, you use high heat and the risk for these cancer-related chemicals to develop goes up, but we don't typically cook vegetables in this way. Bottom line: skip the hot dogs and bacon and opt for some healthier foods, like spinach.

. . . .

For a great way to start your day with spinach, check out the Garlicky Spinach Omelet with Sweet Potato Mash. You can also add raw spinach to any smoothie or use it in place of the mixed lettuce in the

Mixed Green Salad with Fertility-Boosting Nutty-Basil Vinaigrette (see page 76). If you're tired of salads, spinach can be a part of other dishes, as well. Make it part of your main meal with the Asian-Spiced Pork Spare Ribs over Sautéed Spinach.

Garlicky Spinach Omelet with Sweet Potato Mash

Eggs are great for any meal, but especially breakfast since they are filling (goodbye to snacking!) and provide a good source of baby-building protein. Spinach is the star ingredient in this dish because it is full of the essential fertility-boosting mineral folate, and the sweet potato adds antioxidants, B vitamins, and Vitamin C.

Makes 2 servings.

1	large sweet potato
4	large eggs
1 tablespoon	olive oil
1 large clove	garlic, diced
1 cup	fresh baby spinach
½ teaspoon	cumin
¼ teaspoon	paprika
	salt and pepper to taste

Start by heating a pot of water, peel and chop the sweet potato into small chunks, and place the sweet potato in the water. Let the water boil until the sweet potato is cooked through, about 5 to 10 minutes (depending on size of the chunks). While the potato is cooking, crack the eggs into a bowl, season with salt, and whisk together until well mixed. Set aside. Heat a sauté pan with the oil over medium heat. Add the garlic and baby spinach, stirring until the spinach starts to wilt. Turn down the heat if the garlic is starting to burn or turning dark brown. Add the eggs to the pan, stir in the spinach and garlic, and let cook for about 3 or so minutes. Use a spatula to flip the egg and continue cooking another 3 minutes (or until egg is cooked through). Turn off the heat and set aside once ready. Drain the sweet potatoes and keep them in the pot, adding the paprika, cumin, salt, and pepper. Mash the sweet potato and serve alongside the omelet.

Asian-Spiced Pork Spare Ribs over Sautéed Spinach

Browning the meat might seem like an unnecessary step, but it helps to seal in the flavor and is well worth the extra effort. This dish is a great option for a weeknight meal, as you can set it up in the slow cooker in the morning and have it ready to go for dinnertime. The spinach is a great alternative to rice, and helps to boost your intake of fertility-friendly folate, magnesium, and vitamin A.

Makes 4 servings.

3 teaspoons	olive oil (save 1 teaspoon for the spinach)
3 pounds	bone-in country style pork spare ribs
¼ cup	low-sodium soy sauce
⅓ cup	orange marmalade
2–3 dashes	cayenne pepper
4 tablespoons	ketchup
4 cloves	garlic, minced (save 1 minced clove for spinach)
1 teaspoon	cumin
1 teaspoon	ground ginger
¼ cup	fresh cilantro, chopped
1	(10–14 ounce) package spinach

Add two teaspoons of olive oil to a pan and over medium-high heat, brown ribs on both sides (2–3 min each). Set aside. In a small bowl, combine the soy sauce, marmalade, cayenne, ketchup, three cloves of minced garlic, cumin, ginger, and cilantro. Pour half into a slow cooker. Top with ribs, and drizzle the ribs with the remaining sauce. Cover and cook on low for 6–8 hours or until meat is tender.

When you are ready to serve the ribs, add remaining teaspoon of olive oil to a pan. Heat over medium heat, and add remaining garlic. Sauté garlic for 1–2 minutes, and then reduce heat to low and add spinach in handfuls. As it cooks down, add more spinach, stirring as you go. Once all spinach has been cooked down, serve alongside the ribs.

• •

There are two important facts to keep in mind about spinach:

1. Even though spinach is an excellent source of calcium, it is not absorbed very well due to the presence of oxalic acid, so don't rely on this food for your calcium.

2. If financially feasible, opt for fresh *organic* spinach. When tested, conventional spinach is found to have more pesticide residues by weight compared to other produce. If fresh organic spinach is too pricey, purchase the frozen organic kind. It's just as nutritious, but likely a lot cheaper!

• •

Fertility-Boosting Food: Papaya

This sweet tropical fruit is an excellent source of vitamins A and C, folate, and fiber. Specific antioxidants called carotenoids are also found in papayas and likely play an important role in fertility. In women with no history of infertility, those with higher blood levels of alpha carotene before conception had a shorter time to pregnancy compared to those with lower levels. Since oxidative stress in ovarian cells (called oocytes) negatively impacts pregnancy, carotenoids, specifically beta-carotene, may help reduce free radicals within these cells. One animal study found that treatment with beta-carotene helped improve the quality of the ovarian cells by combating oxidation. In fact, both animal and human studies show that carotenoids play a particularly important role in hormonal function, obesity, metabolic syndrome, and fat metabolism. Another great thing about papaya is that you don't necessarily need to purchase organic to avoid pesticides. When last tested, papaya made the list of produce that had minimal pesticide residues (however, if you are trying to avoid

GMOs, you may need to opt for organic, because much of the papaya grown in Hawaii is grown with GMO seeds. There is more on GMOs and whether you should be avoiding them coming up in chapter 8).

◆ ◆ ◆

If you've never had papaya, there's no better time than now to start incorporating it into your diet. If it's not in season, pick up a bag of frozen papaya to throw into the Protein-Packed Papaya and Raspberry Breakfast Smoothie for an extra hint of sweetness to complement the berries. If you find this fruit too sweet on its own, make it slightly savory by adding it as a side to any grilled chicken or a shrimp dish.

Protein-Packed Papaya and Raspberry Breakfast Smoothie

This quick-and-easy breakfast drink is a great way to get your vitamin C, folate, fiber, and antioxidants. With the added protein, you've got yourself a meal in a minute.

Makes 1 serving.

2 cups	diced, frozen papaya
1 cup	frozen raspberries
1 cup	oat milk
2 scoops	(or the equivalent of 1 serving) unflavored protein powder
	juice from ½ lime

Combine all ingredients into a blender and pulse until smooth. Serve immediately.

Fertility-Boosting Food: Collard Greens

Collard greens come from the same family of vegetables as kale, broccoli, and cabbage. Collards are a culinary staple in Southern states, but hopefully no matter where you live, collard greens make their way into your kitchen as well. These thick leafy greens provide a plethora of nutrients, including vitamin A, magnesium, and vitamin K, as well as folate. Just 1 cup of cooked collard greens delivers almost ⅓ of your daily amount of folate and calcium and contains more than 2 milligrams of iron and over ⅓ of your daily recommended dose of vitamin C, which will help to absorb the nonheme iron. In addition, collards are rich in vitamin A and beta-carotene, provide half of your daily manganese, have tons of vitamin K (the same cup of cooked collards has over 770 micrograms of vitamin K), and are moderate in choline, pantothenic acid, zinc, potassium, phosphorus, and magnesium. You can easily add collards (either fresh or cooked) as a side to almost any main dish, and especially to meat, poultry, and fish entrées—the iron present in meat will further increase the amount you absorb from the collards (in addition to the vitamin C present in collards, which also aids in iron absorption), upping your overall iron stores at this time. If you're not a meat eater, you can still enjoy the benefits of this nutritious vegetable. In fact, one of the beauties of this food is that you don't have to cook it at all. Swap in chopped collards for any salad base and toss it with a flavorful dressing, shaved cheese, and a handful of nuts. Since folate isn't too stable when heated, eating raw sources of folate rich foods, like collards, is preferred. Plus, folate from food is better absorbed than folic acid from supplements, so a collard green salad is your best bet. Try the Roasted Chicken with Garlicky Kidney Beans and Collards for a hearty meal that is nutritious and easy to prepare. Also, the Mediterranean Scramble is delish!

Healthful Hint

Collards are usually available in supermarkets throughout the United States (not just in the South) year-round, but if you can't get them fresh, frozen ones are just as good (as they're picked at their prime and frozen immediately, which preserves all the nutrients).

Roasted Chicken with Garlicky Kidney Beans and Collards

This dish is a complete meal, and contains many baby-boosting nutrients from the combination of chicken, kidney beans, and collard greens. Kidney beans are an excellent source of fiber and folate and are a non-animal protein source. Use a store-bought rotisserie chicken to save some time in the kitchen, or roast your own.

Makes 4 servings.

1	(10-ounce) box of frozen collard greens (chopped, thawed and drained), or 3½ cups chopped fresh
1	(15-ounce) can kidney beans, drained and rinsed
½ cup	tomato sauce or tomato-based pasta sauce
½ teaspoon	garlic powder
½ teaspoon	onion powder
1 tablespoon	hot sauce
1	store-bought rotisserie chicken

Combine the collard greens, kidney beans, tomato sauce, garlic powder, onion powder, and hot sauce in a medium skillet and cook over medium-low heat for 10 minutes. Serve on top of sliced chicken.

Mediterranean Scramble

Give your soon-to-be little one all the nutrients and fuel they need to develop and grow inside you with this mixture. The eggs alone are an important source of vitamin B_{12} and choline, both of which are essential for proper nervous system development happening before you will even know if you are pregnant. With additional sources of healthy fats (from the olive oil and olives), and plenty of micronutrients, antioxidants, and phytonutrients, this egg scramble is the perfect way to start your day.

Makes 2 servings.

2 tablespoons	extra-virgin olive oil
4	eggs
½ cup	white button mushrooms, chopped
2 tablespoons	sun-dried tomatoes, chopped
2 cups	fresh collard greens, chopped
4	kalamata olives, chopped
1 tablespoon	balsamic vinegar

Heat the olive oil in a skillet over medium heat. Add the eggs, mushrooms, and sun-dried tomatoes. Stir to mix and cook for about 2 minutes, or until eggs are cooked through. Divide the eggs onto two plates. Add the collard greens, and sprinkle balsamic vinegar and chopped kalamata olives on top.

Healthful Hint

Kidney beans can be a great staple food to keep on hand. Because fiber helps decrease the speed of digestion, the fiber content in foods like kidney beans helps keep your blood glucose (blood sugar) levels from spiking. This is good news for keeping your insulin levels in check, because high levels of insulin decrease the rate of implantation. Besides their stellar nutritional composition, what's great about kidney beans is that they are large and have a good texture. They taste delicious in stews and as a replacement for ground beef in chili. Swapping out meat for beans in your chili would add lots of bioactive compounds, including phytates and phenols, that play important roles related to metabolism in our body. Plus, by subbing kidney beans for ground beef, you basically just eliminated the saturated fat!

Fertility-Boosting Food: Pumpkin Seeds

Pumpkin seeds are an excellent source of zinc, magnesium, and iron, as well as vitamin E and polyunsaturated fatty acids (PUFAs), providing both omega-3 and omega-6 fatty acids. Plus, if you're trying to increase your protein and iron from non-animal sources, pumpkin seeds are perfect. Just one serving of pumpkin seeds (which is about 3 tablespoons) has 7 grams of protein, and over 20 percent of your daily iron needs (not to mention over 30 percent of phosphorus and magnesium needs). Pumpkin seeds also contain numerous compounds, including phenolic acids and carotenoids. The extracts from these little seeds have been shown to have blood-sugar-lowering properties and anticancer benefits, and they also play a role in reproductive health due to certain phytoestrogens. For all of these reasons, pumpkin seeds are a great addition to a homemade trail mix, taste great in Greek yogurt for an added crunchy texture, and they make a great snack on their own. For a healthy breakfast option, swap in pumpkin seeds instead of the sunflower seeds in the Cashew and Pomegranate Granola Cereal on page 81. Or, if you are looking for a go-to snack that can keep you feeling energized and help improve your fertility, try the No-Bake Nut-Free Granola Bites with Honey and Lavender, which uses pumpkin seeds in place of nuts.

No-Bake Nut-Free Granola Bites with Honey and Lavender

Granola bites make a healthy snack, and making your own is not hard. This nut-free and no-bake version uses pumpkin seeds for extra zinc, magnesium, and healthy omega-3 and omega-6 fatty acids. Use this as your go-to snack when on the run.

Makes about 12 bites.

1 cup	old-fashioned oats
3 tablespoons	culinary lavender (ground)
½ cup	pumpkin seeds

½ cup   sunflower butter
2 teaspoons brown sugar
⅓ cup   honey
1 teaspoon   vanilla extract
1 teaspoon   cinnamon

Mix oats, lavender, pumpkin seeds, sunflower butter, brown sugar, honey, vanilla and cinnamon in a bowl until well combined. Chill in the refrigerator for at least 1 hour. Form into small (2-inch) balls. Store in an airtight container for 1 week.

Fertility-Boosting Food: Chickpeas

Chickpeas, or garbanzo beans, are versatile legumes packed with micronutrients needed to help support a healthy pregnancy including iron, potassium, and selenium. They are also a great meat protein alternative, providing almost 15 grams of protein per cup. Plus, we digest the protein in chickpeas well, as it scores pretty high on the protein digestibility scale. They are also an excellent source of soluble fiber. Since fiber slows digestion, it helps you feel fuller for longer while also benefiting your gut microbes. The good news is that canned chickpeas retain their nutritional value, so if you're short on time, you don't need to worry about soaking the dried ones. Just make sure that you purchase a bisphenol A (BPA)–free lined can and rinse the beans under cold water to help remove a lot of the extra sodium (see chapter 8 for more on why BPA should be avoided when trying to conceive). Importantly, chickpeas are also rich in vitamin B_6. This coenzyme is involved in multiple reactions in our body and has been shown to increase the chance of conception in women who were subfertile as well as decreasing the chance of a miscarriage.

Chickpeas are a main ingredient in the Spicy Tuna and Chickpea Salad Sandwich or the Turkey-Prosciutto Club With Homemade Chickpea Spread. If you're in the mood for a chickpea snack, whip up some creamy Homemade Lemon Hummus (see page 74) for a treat rich in vitamin B_6. Or, if you are looking for an easy weeknight meal, try the Spicy Canned Salmon with Chickpea Salad Cups on page 103.

Spicy Tuna and Chickpea Salad Sandwich

This dish may have a lot of ingredients, but it's actually super simple, and you can easily make extra tuna salad to set aside in the refrigerator for later. This recipe has everything you need to support your fertility diet plan, including lean protein, fiber, omega-3s, vitamin A, B vitamins, vitamin C, vitamin D, iron, selenium, phytonutrients, and much more. Make sure to store the almonds and tuna salad mixture separately to keep the almonds from getting soggy.

Makes 4 sandwiches.

1	(15-ounce) can chickpeas (no sodium added)
1	lemon, juiced
1	(5-ounce) can chunk light tuna, packed in water
1	avocado, peeled and pitted
½ cup	shredded carrot
2 stalks	celery, finely chopped
½	red onion, finely chopped
1 tablespoon	fresh dill
2 teaspoons	sriracha
⅛ teaspoon	cayenne pepper
	salt and pepper to taste
⅓ cup	slivered almonds
8 slices	whole-grain bread
1 cup	arugula

Drain and rinse the chickpeas and place them in a mixing bowl. Add the juice of one lemon and use a fork or other utensil to mash up the chickpeas. Drain the tuna and add to the bowl along with the avocado, carrot, celery, onion, dill, sriracha, cayenne, salt, and pepper, mixing everything together. To plate, add a fist-size portion of the mixture onto one slice of bread, flatten out, and add slivered almonds and arugula on top. Close the sandwich with another piece of bread.

Turkey-Prosciutto Club with Homemade Chickpea Spread

This hearty sandwich is a meal in itself. The chickpea spread is a healthy alternative to traditional condiments, giving you added nutrients and protein.

Makes 4 sandwiches.

1	(15-ounce) can chickpeas
1 stalk	celery, chopped
1 tablespoon	mayonnaise
1 tablespoon	fresh dill, chopped
1 tablespoon	lemon juice
8 slices	whole-grain bread, toasted
4–6 slices	fresh turkey breast (not deli meat, buy a fresh pre-cooked turkey breast)
¼ pound	sliced prosciutto
4–5 leaves	Bibb lettuce

To make the chickpea spread, mash chickpeas in a medium-sized bowl with a fork. Add celery, mayonnaise, dill, and lemon juice, and mix to combine. Set aside. To plate, spread the chickpea spread on one side of the toast. Top with turkey, then prosciutto, and lettuce. Smear another piece of toast with the chickpea spread and close the sandwich.

Fertility-Boosting Food: Lentils

Lentils are loaded with folate and another great example of a plant-based protein. Only ½ cup of cooked lentils provides 12 g of protein. Also, early on in pregnancy (before you will likely even be able to know if you are pregnant) folate is key, and lentils are simply packed with it! In addition, they're a good source of iron to start building up your stores from the very beginning. They are packed with fiber, resistance starch, and prebiotics, all of which help keep your blood sugar levels from spiking and keep your gut health in check. Lentils also contain vitamin B_6, potassium, and zinc, among other things. Lentils are also a great source of polyphenols, further supporting their protective role in diabetes and inflammation, which are two conditions that negatively impact pregnancy.

Lentils are also high in several minerals needed to support reproductive health, including copper, phosphorus, manganese, and iron. Since they don't need to be soaked first, they are easier to cook from scratch (compared to other beans), and they don't take very long to prepare. Pair them with a whole grain, and you have a complete protein. Or, you can just add them to a salad or soup as an easy way to up your meal's nutritional value. For a delicious dish that is hearty and nutritious, try the Chicken Curry and Lentil Soup with Toasted Ciabatta.

Chicken Curry and Lentil Soup with Toasted Ciabatta

Folate- and fiber-packed lentils make this delicious soup hearty and healthy. The flavors of the chicken, curry and coconut combine to make this a fragrant dish that is great for dinner.

Makes 6 servings.

1 tablespoon	canola oil
1	large onion, diced
3 cloves	garlic, minced
3 tablespoons	curry powder
½ cup	uncooked lentils
1 pound	chicken breast, grilled and shredded with a fork
4 cups	reduced sodium chicken broth
3 cups	water
1 cup	coconut milk
6 slices	ciabatta bread, toasted
	finely chopped fresh cilantro, for garnish

Heat oil in Dutch oven over low heat. Add onion and garlic and cook while stirring for about 5 minutes. Add curry powder and lentils and cook 5 more minutes. Add chicken broth and water. Bring to a boil. Reduce heat to simmer and cook for 30 minutes. Remove from heat, and in batches puree in a blender. Return soup to Dutch oven, and add shredded chicken and coconut milk, and cook for 5 minutes. Serve with cilantro as garnish on soup along with sliced ciabatta.

Fertility-Boosting Food: Canned Tuna Fish

Contrary to popular belief, not all tuna needs to be avoided prior to and during pregnancy. While you do want to limit albacore tuna (solid/chunk white) to once a week, canned light tuna is actually a good way to increase the amount of fish you eat while avoiding high intakes of mercury. Like other animal proteins, tuna is an excellent source of protein. However, studies have shown that unlike other meats, fish intake is associated with a shorter time to pregnancy. It's likely a combination of the essential fatty acids, vitamin D, and minerals like selenium that make fish so favorable for fertility. Selenium in particular is a key mineral, and it also may have a protective effect on mercury exposure.

Overall, canned light tuna is an easy way to get more fish in your diet, which may improve your odds of conceiving. Plus, research shows that higher fish intake compared to other meats is associated with better semen quality and improves chances of live birth in women undergoing IVF treatment.

You can enjoy canned tuna with some lemon juice on a green salad for an easy lunch, or try the Grilled Three-Cheese Tuna Melt Sandwich with Chicken Noodle Soup for a "diner style" tuna melt. Or simply follow the recipe for the Fertility-Friendly "Sushi" Bowl (page 70) or the Spicy Tuna and Chickpea Salad Sandwich (page 96).

Grilled Three-Cheese Tuna Melt Sandwich with Chicken Noodle Soup

This pairing of the classic tuna melt with chicken noodle soup is a hearty and healthy dinner. It contains fertility-boosting nutrients such as omega-3 fatty acids and selenium from the tuna and calcium from the cheese. Sandwiches don't store well, but soup does, so this recipe makes for extra soup that you can enjoy later on or freeze for up to 3 months.

Makes approximately 10 servings of soup and 2 servings of sandwiches.

FOR THE SOUP

5 cups	chicken stock
8 cups	water
4	chicken thighs, boneless
2 tablespoons	olive oil
1	medium yellow onion, chopped
3	celery stalks, chopped
3	carrots, sliced into coins
½ pound	pasta (rotini or cavatappi work best)
1 clove	garlic, minced
1 teaspoon	salt
½ teaspoon	pepper

FOR THE SANDWICH

2 tablespoons	butter
1	(5-ounce) can chunk light tuna, packed in water
4 slices	whole-grain bread
2 slices	mozzarella cheese
2 slices	yellow sharp cheddar cheese
2 slices	Gouda cheese

To prepare the soup, in a large pot, combine water and chicken stock. Bring to a boil, and add chicken thighs. Boil for about 20 minutes, and skim off any foam that forms on the surface.

While the chicken is cooking, add olive to a skillet over medium heat, and sauté onion, celery, and carrots for about 7 minutes, or until softened. Add to pot. Add pasta to pot, and cook for another 10 minutes. While pasta is cooking, remove the chicken and use a fork to shred it into smaller pieces. Return it to the pot. Add salt, pepper, and garlic.

To prepare the sandwiches, heat a griddle pan over medium heat. Butter the tops of bread, and place 2 slices buttered-side-down on griddle. Add a slice of cheese to the bread, and then add ½ can of tuna. Top tuna with slices of the other cheeses, and top with another slice of buttered bread, with butter facing up. Cook for 3–4 minutes, then flip and cook for another 3 minutes, until bread is toasted and cheese is melted.

Serve soup alongside the sandwich.

• •

Are All Canned Tunas Safe?

Canned tuna can contain mercury, but some contains more than others. Albacore tuna is known to have a higher mercury content, so opt for other varieties, such as chunk light.

• •

Fertility-Boosting Food: Salmon

Salmon is both a nutrient- and energy-dense fish. This fish is rich in omega-3 fatty acids, selenium, and vitamin D, as well as B_{12}. The fatty acids that are abundant in salmon are protective against cardio-vascular disease, depression, and infertility! In fact, fats are actually consistently shown to be the most tied to fertility health compared to other nutrients. Plus, omega-3s are vital for the brain health, nervous system development, and the cognition of your baby-to-be! Another good thing about salmon when compared to other fish is that it is lower in mercury, which is something to always be mindful about (especially before conception and during pregnancy).

Salmon comes fresh, frozen, or canned, but try to avoid farmed salmon. When compared to wild-caught salmon, farmed salmon has been shown to have more saturated fat and high levels of contaminants that can be toxic. Wild salmon is typically a little more expensive than farmed, but canned wild salmon is a great alternative. It is a really easy and inexpensive way to get your dose of omega-3s without breaking the bank. Plus, just a 3-ounce can provides close to half of your selenium needs and is loaded with vitamin D! Check out the recipe for Salmon and Yukon Gold Potato Hash. Or for a quick but nutritious lunch, try the Spicy Canned Salmon with Chickpea Salad Cups.

Salmon and Yukon Gold Potato Hash

All you really need for this dish is some salmon, potatoes, and your favorite herbs for a quick, easy, fertility-boosting dinner. Salmon is an excellent source of omega-3 fatty acids, which help increase your chances of getting pregnant. Not to mention this is a great recipe to have on hand once you get pregnant, since omega-3s are essential to proper brain development in a fetus.

Makes about 4 servings.

4 tablespoons	unsalted butter or olive oil
1½–2 pounds	Yukon Gold potatoes, diced
1	yellow onion, diced
2 stalks	celery, diced
1 tablespoon	fresh dill, chopped
2 teaspoons	fresh thyme, minced
	salt and pepper to taste
1 pound	cooked, flaked salmon
½ cup	parsley, chopped
	hot sauce for serving, optional

In a large frying pan, heat the butter or oil over medium heat. Add the potatoes and onions, sauté for about 1 minute until coated with butter or oil, then cover the pan to steam the potatoes for about 6 to 8 minutes. The potatoes should be almost tender. Add the celery and stir, then cover again for 2 minutes. Uncover the pan and add the dill, thyme, and salt and pepper to taste. Continue to cook the potatoes and herbs for about 15 more minutes, stirring occasionally, until lightly browned. Finally, add the cooked salmon and parsley and cook just until the salmon is heated through. Overcooking may leave the salmon dry and chewy. Serve immediately.

Spicy Canned Salmon with Chickpea Salad Cups

Canned salmon is an easy, cheap, and excellent source of fertility-promoting protein and both EPA and DHA omega-3 fatty acids. This spicy dish can be adjusted accordingly to your taste preferences.

Makes 2 servings.

1 can	wild salmon
1	avocado
½	lemon, juiced
⅛ teaspoon	cayenne pepper
1 cup	canned chickpeas (make sure can is BPA free)
¼ cup	scallions, chopped
½	cucumber, finely chopped
	sea salt and pepper to taste
4 leaves	romaine (or Bibb lettuce)

In a mixing bowl, mash the avocado together with the canned salmon, lemon juice, and cayenne. Mix in the chickpeas, scallions, and cucumber. Season with sea salt and pepper to taste. Divide the salmon salad between the romaine leaves.

Fertility-Boosting Food: Chicken

Chicken is a good source of heme iron (the iron type that is more readily absorbed) and high-biological-value protein, both of which are needed to support a healthy pregnancy. Iron is needed to make hormones for growth, and the amount that you need during pregnancy increases, so it's a good thing to make sure you're not lacking prior to pregnancy. Adequate protein is also necessary, and lean meat chicken provides 30 grams in only 4 ounces. That same amount also delivers 1.2 mg of iron. Just remember to remove the skin to keep it lean!

Chicken is far less controversial when compared to red and processed meats when considering overall health and disease. Since high intakes of red and processed meats are associated with increased risk of multiple comorbid conditions and negative fertility outcomes, leaner protein sources like chicken are likely to be a better option. Further, it's also a great source of choline and vitamin B$_6$, as well as phosphorus and zinc.

Chicken can be prepared so many different ways, but avoid frying it. Try the Grilled Chicken Salad Rolls with Peanut Sauce for lunch, or the Cherry-Glazed Chicken Kebabs for dinner. If you are in the mood for soup, check out the Chicken Curry and Lentil Soup with Toasted Ciabatta (page 98) or the Grilled Three-Cheese Tuna Melt with Chicken Noodle Soup (page 100).

Grilled Chicken Salad Rolls with Peanut Sauce

Chicken is not only versatile and easy to cook but also a great source of lean protein. The red cabbage and carrots are loaded with antioxidants, and the Greek yogurt is a great protein-packed alternative to mayo.

Makes 2 servings.

FOR THE CHICKEN SALAD

	olive oil spray
7–8 ounces	chicken breast
½ cup	reduced-fat Greek yogurt
⅛ cup	finely chopped red onion
½ cup	shredded red cabbage

¼ cup	shredded carrots
1 teaspoon	grated ginger
2 tablespoons	chopped cilantro
squeeze	lime juice
	whole wheat wrap or large romaine lettuce leaves

FOR THE PEANUT SAUCE

2 tablespoons	smooth peanut butter
1 teaspoon	low-sodium soy sauce
1 teaspoon	honey or agave syrup
1 teaspoon	water
1 teaspoon	chopped garlic
	squeeze fresh lime juice

Spray grill or oven pan with olive oil spray and cook chicken until completely cooked through (interior temperature of 165° F). In a large bowl, mix together the yogurt, onion, cabbage, carrots, ginger, cilantro, and a squeeze of lime juice. Once the chicken has cooled enough to handle, cut into smaller pieces and incorporate into mixture. To prepare the peanut sauce, add peanut butter, soy sauce, honey, water, garlic, and a squeeze of lime juice to a bowl and whisk together until incorporated. If you want the sauce a little spicy, add in some crushed red pepper or chili flakes. Place the chicken mixture into wraps or lettuce and roll up. Serve with peanut sauce for dipping, or drizzle it on top before serving.

Cherry-Glazed Chicken Kebabs

When you want barbecue but don't feel like having beef, these kebabs are a great alternative. The chicken is a source of protein and iron, and the veggies give you extra nutrients. Cherries are rich in polyphenols and good sources of antioxidants like vitamin C. Since cherries are naturally sweet, you won't need any added sugar for this dish.

Makes 4 kebabs.

1 tablespoon	olive oil
3 tablespoons	minced shallots
1 clove	garlic, minced
¾ cup	cherry preserves (look for a low-sugar or sugar-free version)
¼ cup	balsamic vinegar
⅛ teaspoon	ground pepper
4	wooden skewers (presoaked in water)
4	chicken breasts, cut into 1-inch cubes
1	green bell pepper, cut into 1-inch pieces
1	red bell pepper, cut into 1-inch pieces
½	medium onion, cut into wedges
1	medium zucchini, cut into coins
8	cherry tomatoes

In a medium saucepan, heat the olive oil over medium heat. Add shallots and garlic and sauté for about 3 minutes. Add cherry preserves, balsamic vinegar and ground pepper. Reduce heat to low and cook until mixture has reduced, approximately 8 minutes. Set glaze aside.

Assemble kebabs by taking skewers and adding green pepper, chicken, red pepper, onion, and zucchini, in that pattern, until skewer is full. Cap kebab with a cherry tomato on each end. Heat the grill to medium-high heat. Brush glaze on the kebabs, and grill until chicken is well done, approximately 4 minutes per side. As you rotate the kebabs, brush with more glaze.

◆ ◆ ◆

Now what?

I bet now you have a ton of ideas for what to eat, but sometimes too much information can be overwhelming. Not to worry, as in chapter 7 I am going to show you some meal plans to help you get organized with eating the *right* foods to boost your fertility. But first, we need to go over some of the foods that you should be *avoiding or limiting*, as they can be harmful to your reproductive health and fertility.

CHAPTER 6

Twenty Foods You Should Avoid (or Limit) When You Want to Get Pregnant

We have been talking a lot about the type of nutrients that can help improve your fertility, and which foods contain them. In the previous chapter, we reviewed twenty foods that can help to boost your fertility, along with several ideas to incorporate them into your diet. While incorporating these foods into your diet is a great way to help improve your chances of getting pregnant, we also must address some foods that you should avoid or limit, as studies suggest that they can hinder your chances of conceiving, for a variety of reasons that we will go over next.

Now, I don't want you to freak out if you have been eating these foods. I am in no way saying that it is your fault that you aren't pregnant because you have been eating these foods. Many of them are thought to be healthy, and for people who aren't trying to get pregnant, they often can be. But for those who are trying to get pregnant, these foods can have specific effects on our health that can, in some cases, hinder the process.

Some of these foods may shock you. Who would have thought kale or grapes, which are thought to be the epitome of healthy foods, could impede fertility? You will find out why in this chapter.

Fertility-Reducing Food: Juice

Juice is often thought of as "healthy" and a better alternative to other sweet beverages like soda or lemonade, but most juices aren't much lower in sugar or calories. For example, one 8-ounce cup of apple juice provides the same amount of sugar as 8 ounces of certain colas. Don't let the labels fool you; even if the juice reads "no sugar added" on the label, there is still a lot of sugar naturally present in juice. This is why even fresh pressed juices are not great options either.

High intake of sugar is associated with negative fertility outcomes in men and women, and avoiding it will prevent exaggerated hormonal fluctuations and will help keep inflammation at bay. Also, sugar-sweetened beverages, like fruit juice, have been linked to obesity, cardiovascular disease, and also increased mortality risk (yikes!). Even if you weren't trying to get pregnant, you should avoid them for these reasons!

Besides the fact that juice is calorically dense and nutrient poor, some are contaminated with heavy metals like arsenic and lead, which are known to be associated with poorer reproductive health. Women with higher levels of lead had significantly more uterine fibroids when compared to those without elevated levels. Moreover, higher levels of lead and arsenic have been associated with infertility, preeclampsia, and miscarriage (there is more information on these toxic metals in chapter 8). So, in addition to all of the sugar you're saving from passing on the juice, you are also avoiding unwanted metal ingestion.

If you're nervous you are missing out on vitamin C, grab an actual orange instead of orange juice. One orange is about 15 grams of sugar and 3 grams of fiber, compared to juice, which has twice the amount of sugar and no fiber at all.

. . . .

Healthful Hint

Instead of juice, go for the smoothie. When you blend the entire fruit, you are getting all of the nutrients and fiber that are contained in the fruit, not just the sugar.

. . . .

Fertility-Reducing Food: Blackened Salmon

Eating salmon is an excellent way to increase your fish (and omega-3 fatty acid) intake while limiting your mercury exposure, but the way it's prepared may be hurting your chances of getting pregnant. When foods are blackened and charred, different chemicals are created due to the high-temperature cooking. Some of the chemicals that are formed have been associated with increased cancer risk as well as infertility.

Although the spices added to blackened fish add some nutritional value compared to fried or battered fish, the chemicals that are formed from the high heat contribute to inflammation and interfere with your endocrine system. Formation of acrylamide, advanced glycated end products (AGEs), and polycyclic aromatic hydrocarbons (PAH) occur when foods are cooked with high heat. Animal proteins that are higher in fat, such as salmon, produce more AGEs than other foods (like vegetables) when heated. Beside higher levels of AGEs, the PAHs are also detrimental. Not only are they carcinogenic, but exposure has been associated with early pregnancy loss. Instead of having your salmon prepared on the grill, use a moist heat method of cooking and add an acidic marinade or spices (both have been shown to decrease the amount of AGEs produced when compared to alternative high-heat cooking) so you can still enjoy a healthy piece of fish without the worry.

Fertility-Reducing Food: Canned Fruit (in Syrup or Juice)

If purchasing fresh fruit is not always feasible, think twice before replacing it with the canned variety. Not to say that all canned fruit is "bad," but it's important to read the labels, because not all canned fruit is created equal.

Many types are sitting in juice or heavy syrup, adding a lot more sugar and calories to what could be a healthy snack. Certain varieties also contain artificial colors, stabilizers, and flavoring agents. Plus, there's a high probability that the BPA from the can lining leached into the fruit. In fact, when testing urine BPA concentration levels, researchers found that there was 70 percent more BPA present in those who ate one can or more as compared to people who did not eat canned fruit. If you are looking for a healthier alternative, opt for canned fruit that is packed in water, with no sugar added.

• •

What is BPA?

Bisphenol A is a synthetic chemical that is found in many food storage products. It is discussed in greater detail in chapter 8, so flip ahead to read more about why this can be bad for you when trying to conceive.

If fresh fruit isn't an option, try frozen. With frozen fruit you won't have to worry about BPA. Plus, frozen fruit retains more of its vitamins and phenolic compounds when compared to many canned varieties.

• •

Fertility-Reducing Food: Alcohol

Although we don't typically think of it as one, alcohol is a food because it contains calories. If you aren't someone who typically drinks alcohol, giving it up won't be a problem for you. However, if you do drink alcohol, it may be a good idea to limit your total intake. But first, let's review how much a standard drink is:

12 ounces of regular beer = 5 ounces of wine = 1.5 ounces of liquor

Although the research on alcohol and fertility continues to be inconclusive, alcohol in general is not considered "healthy." While a beer or occasional glass of wine won't harm you, when consumed regularly, any possible benefits of alcohol are negated by the health risks it poses. Not only is it energy dense with virtually no micronutrients, it is also associated with increased risk of many diseases, including cancer. Further, alcohol does impact hormone levels and can negatively affect the cells that become an embryo and actual implantation. While low to moderate alcohol intake may not negatively impact fertility or be as "bad" as once thought, one study found that women who reported drinking more than seven drinks per week (think a little more than a glass of wine each night) have a significantly longer time conceiving when compared to women who drink less. Overall, the relationship between alcohol and fertility remains to be debated. However, many women don't realize they are pregnant until a couple of weeks in, and no amount of alcohol is considered to be "safe" during pregnancy. So if you're actively trying to conceive, avoiding it is recommended.

Fertility-Reducing Food: Regular Soda

Soda is always on the list of unhealthy foods and beverages because of its high sugar content. It is also associated with many different disease states. Soda intake is not only damaging to your liver and your heart, but it also is associated with infertility. One study found that women who reported drinking three or more servings of soda per day had more than a 50 percent lower rate of having a healthy pregnancy compared to women who abstained from soda. But soda isn't detrimental to just women; there appears to be a correlation between soda intake and lower semen quality and infertility in men. In fact, low testosterone levels are shown to be significantly associated with higher intake of sugar-sweetened beverages. In addition to the almost 40 grams of sugar in each can, many sodas contain caffeine. Although the effect that caffeine has on fertility is highly debated, there does seem to be an increased risk of miscarriage with high caffeine intake. We also know that type 2 diabetes, which is a disease related to sugar and sugar metablolism, negatively impacts fertility in males. Plus, all that sugar increases your risk of gestational diabetes and adversely impacts the health of your baby-to-be!

• •

Sugar Is Everywhere

It's naturally found in foods like fruits, vegetables, and legumes, but even more so it's found in a ton of processed foods and drinks. Sodas and sugar-sweetened beverages like sports drinks, energy drinks, and fruit juice are leading sources of added sugar in our diets. A small juice box (6 ounces) of fruit juice can pack 20 grams of sugar, whereas a 12-ounce soda can pack 39 grams. The American Heart Association recommends that you limit added sugar intake to 100 calories a day (25 grams or 6 teaspoons) for women and 150 calories a day (36 grams or 9 teaspoons) for men. That means that drinking just one 12-ounce can of soda has more added sugar than is recommended to have in a whole day.

• •

Unfortunately, there aren't many studies looking at the effects of sugar intake specifically on female fertility. However, we do see increases of infertility in women with type 2 diabetes. Sugar is also associated with a number of other conditions which impact fertility: delayed age of puberty, irregular menstruation, a possible link to polycystic ovary syndrome (PCOS), and a decrease in successful live births, among many other factors.

In order to limit your sugar intake, the best thing you can do is to always opt for whole foods over processed ones. Typically, processed foods and drinks, such as sodas, sports drinks, juices, candy bars, ice cream, baked goods, cereal, yogurt, and even things that are seemingly healthy, like salad dressings or stir-fry sauce contain high amounts of sugar. It is important to be able to read and compare nutrition and ingredient labels of your favorite foods and choose those that are lowest in sugar, especially added sugar. Sources of sugar like honey, maple syrup, agave, coconut sugar, etc., aren't necessarily any healthier than regular table sugar. See page 145 for some tips on how to decipher Nutrition Facts labels so you can be sure that you are keeping your sugar intake in check.

• •

The Many Names of Sugar

Cutting back on sugar is so hard, in part, because it is everywhere. It is in so many foods and beverages that we eat that it can be hard to find sugar-less options. And to make matters even more difficult, sugar goes by about 56 different names! So next time you grab something to eat and it contains agave, fruit concentrate, or brown rice syrup, know that those are all code words for sugar.

• •

Fertility-Reducing Food:
Artificially Sweetened Beverages

If you plan on giving up sugary soda to increase your chances of getting pregnant, don't make the switch to diet just yet. While one study didn't find a negative relationship between diet soda and becoming pregnant, another study found that diet beverage intake *did* negatively impact the health of the oocyte, decreased the quality of the embryo and lowered pregnancy rates in women who were undergoing assisted reproduction. Differences in the quality and actual type of study typically account for differences in findings, but avoiding diet soda is probably a good idea, regardless. Besides the artificial sweetener in all diet sodas, think about the chemicals, and dyes. Plus, many of the food dyes that are used have questionable safety profiles, including being toxic to your cell's genetic material. A study conducted in rats found that one food dye actually decreased sperm count. So if you're looking for a no-calorie beverage, switch to infused waters or seltzers. You'll stay adequately hydrated while avoiding an unnecessary ingestion of chemicals.

• •

Sweet N' Low, Equal, Splenda, and NutraSweet are just some of several artificial sweeteners you may use, or have used at one point to satisfy your sweet tooth without the calories. You may also know these by their chemical names: aspartame, sucralose, saccharin, acesulfame, and neotame. To reduce your intake of artificial sweeteners, it's important to know the names of these products and check the ingredient labels of the products you buy. Artificial sweeteners are commonly found in diet foods and drinks, gum, and foods labeled "low-sugar" or "sugar-free," such as jams, jellies, yogurts, and baked goods.

• •

Fertility-Reducing Food: White Rice

Have you ever ordered takeout and eaten an entire container of white rice, and then within an hour you feel like you can eat again? One reason why you may feel this way is because of the high glycemic load of white rice. Since white rice has been stripped of all of its fiber, your body digests it very quickly, and it doesn't give you the same satiating effects as when you eat a high-fiber grain or even a potato. Besides making you feel hungrier, it also causes a surge in insulin to try and get all that sugar out of your blood. Eating white rice often (as well as other refined carbs) causes chronically high levels of insulin, which can lead to other hormonal changes that can negatively impact fertility outcomes. So go easy on refined carbohydrates like white rice, and swap in higher-fiber varieties or other grains instead. The higher fiber content will help keep your blood sugar levels in a normal range and keep you fuller longer!

Fertility-Reducing Food: Hot Soup (or Beverage) from a Polystyrene Container

Sometimes the culprit for reducing fertility isn't in the food, but in the vessel in which it is contained. We will discuss food containers and packaging in greater detail in chapter 8, but it is good to keep in mind now when thinking about foods to avoid. Polystyrene is a type of plastic that has a variety of different uses, but you may be most familiar with it in the form of Styrofoam. Exposure to polystyrene is associated with respiratory and neurological diseases, as well as cancer and eye problems. Although not currently considered endocrine disruptors, prenatal exposure to polystyrene is detrimental to your growing baby. There is evidence in animals that it harms reproduction, but according to the Environmental Protection Agency, the evidence is inconclusive for humans. However, due to the negative effects exposure has on people and growing babies, it's likely best to avoid it. The good news is that many food retailers have stopped using it and some states have actually banned it, because it is terrible for the environment. However, since it is a trusty temperature insulator, a lot of food establishments do still use it. But beware, because hotter temperatures cause many chemicals from the polystyrene to leach into your food. So if your favorite food retailer still hands you your coffee in a Styrofoam cup, see if they wouldn't mind filling up your own reusable one. If not, ask them for a paper cup instead!

Fertility-Reducing Food: Fast-Food Cheeseburger

Regardless of whether or not you're trying to get pregnant, avoiding fast food is a good idea. Highly processed food from your local fast-food joint is not doing you or your partner's reproductive system, or any system for that matter, any good. Multiple studies show that fast-food intake is associated with worse fertility outcomes. Compared with women who consumed fast food four or more times per week, those who did not had a 41 percent reduced risk of suffering from infertility. Maybe it's the abnormally high fat content of a fast-food cheeseburger that contributes to the decline of fecundity (another word for fertility), or it could also be the extreme amount of advanced glycation end products (AGEs) that those burgers carry. As mentioned earlier, AGEs are naturally present in foods with uncooked animal proteins and fat, but when these proteins and fat are cooked, more AGEs are made. The reaction of sugars with either protein or fat causes more of these chemicals to form, and high heat like frying really accelerates the process. In fact, head-to-head, a burger from a famous fast-food place delivers more than double the AGEs of a burger made at home.

• •

Why Should I Be Concerned About AGEs?

AGEs are associated with multiple diseases like diabetes and kidney disease, and women with PCOS have been found to have naturally higher levels of AGEs in their body. Since AGEs are inflammatory, it's likely that they compromise reproductive health. In fact, higher levels of AGEs in the uteri of women with obesity (compared to lean women) were found to negatively impact endometrial function and may be another explanation for infertility.

• •

So if you're craving a cheeseburger, skip the drive-through and make one at home (with a lower-fat beef, or better yet, ground turkey, and not over a high flame) in order to decrease your intake of these problematic compounds.

Fertility-Reducing Food: Nonorganic Kale

You are probably wondering why on earth the almighty kale is on a list of foods *not* to eat. If you're trying to conceive, kale may not be the best way to go about getting your greens in. Yes, kale is loaded with fiber and micronutrients to support a growing baby, but unfortunately conventional kale made the list of produce with the highest amounts of pesticides. In fact, when different samples of nonorganic kale were tested, there were over 15 different pesticides present. Kale and spinach averaged to have anywhere from 1.1–1.8 times more pesticides than other crops. Since nonorganic fruits and veggies are how most people are exposed to pesticides, trying to avoid ones that make the list of "dirtiest" produce is a good way to decrease the amount that you're taking in. But this doesn't mean you should avoid kale completely! If financially feasible, spring for organic. If fresh organic kale (or spinach) isn't in your budget, try frozen organic kale. Since you can't use frozen kale for a salad, opt for a cleaner green. Cabbage is a great option that doesn't have nearly as many pesticides, and it tastes great shredded as a salad base or even roasted to bring out its natural sweetness.

Fertility-Reducing Food: Bacon

Bacon is just one of the several types of meats you should forgo if you're trying to get pregnant. In fact, your partner should put the bacon down also. Study after study points to processed meats as a main dietary culprit negatively associated with pregnancy. Plus, eating processed meats like bacon is associated with increased risk of problems when you do become pregnant, such a high blood pressure during pregnancy (which can lead to a potentially dangerous pregnancy complication called preeclampsia). One study found that a woman's pre-pregnancy fried-food intake can increase her risk of having gestational diabetes, with higher intakes making the risk even greater. Besides the chemicals that give bacon its pink color and the MSG that helps as a flavor enhancer, the way bacon is typically prepared (fried up in a pan) makes it even worse for our reproductive health. Since bacon (and the like) is associated with many chronic diseases including heart disease and cancer, eating less of it is a good idea for everyone.

Fertility-Reducing Food: Nonorganic Grapes

Although grapes are packed with vitamins and antioxidants, they also deliver a hefty dose of pesticides. When compared to other produce, grapes ranked as one of the highest in contaminants of pesticides. Unfortunately, pesticides do seem to play a role in fertility, and avoiding them is beneficial. Recently a study found that increased adherence to a diet containing lower pesticides increased the likelihood of becoming pregnant. The data on pesticides and pregnancy is mixed, but that may be due to the fact that pesticide laws across countries differ, making the results of these studies difficult to compare.

Besides pesticides, grapes may not be the best choice if you're trying to keep your blood sugar under control. Grapes have a high glycemic index, so compared to other fruits with more fiber, they are digested rather quickly and make your blood sugar shoot up faster. Don't switch out the grapes for cake though! Grapes are still significantly healthier than junk food, but may not be the best option, especially if they aren't organic. Two conventional fruits that have significantly less pesticides are cantaloupe and kiwis. In fact, over 70 percent of the "cleaner" produce tested had no pesticides on them at all.

• •

Healthful Hint

Melons or other fruits with a thick rind can be a better alternative because they tend to retain less pesticide residue than thin-skinned fruits. If you choose to have melon, make sure to wash the outer layer of all melons before cutting them open. Otherwise, the bacteria on the rind will go into the melon as you slice it up, and this bacteria can be harmful to a growing baby.

• •

Fertility-Reducing Food: Sausage

Whether it's homemade or store bought, sausage isn't doing your reproductive health any good. Yes, store-bought sausage will likely have a very long list of chemicals that you can't pronounce that homemade sausage won't, but either way it's a good idea to limit how much of it you eat when you're trying to become pregnant. Since too much red and processed meat intake is associated with worse fertility outcomes in both men and women, swapping out sausage links for a piece of fish or leaner protein source is desirable. One study found that when switching out red or processed meat for fish, chances of having a successful pregnancy significantly increased. Plus, sausage is loaded with fat, and just one link can have over 15 grams! Not only is this not good for your heart, but women who eat a high-fat diet may have a reduced ability to become pregnant. Plus, less meat has been shown to benefit embryonic growth!

If you are going to have a sausage link, bake it in the oven (with some peppers for a kick of vitamin C) instead of over a high flame on the grill (to help reduce some of the chemicals that are formed at very high heat). And opt for sausages that are made with lean cuts of meat or poultry to decrease your total fat intake.

Fertility-Reducing Food: Canned Creamy Tomato Soup

As you know, diet can either help or hurt your chances of becoming pregnant, and unfortunately, as we have discussed previously, so can the containers that food comes in. There are a lot of good things about canned foods. Not only are they are a cost-effective way to get healthful foods, but they have a long shelf life and are super convenient. However, there are some negatives that come along with eating canned foods. Just like water bottles, most cans are lined with BPA, a known endocrine disruptor associated with fertility issues. Since many consumers are starting to avoid BPA, companies now make "BPA-free" cans, but those may not be any better because what's used in place of BPA may have very similar effects on our hormones. Canned creamy tomato soup may be even worse than other types of canned food due to its acidity and higher fat content. Plus, canned soups are typically very salty. For example, one can of condensed creamy tomato soup contains over 2000 mg of sodium! That is almost an entire day's worth of suggested sodium intake in just one meal! The fat, salt, and acidity of this soup in particular is more problematic than other canned foods. When a canned food is fatty, acidic, and salty, such as creamy tomato soup, more chemicals will leach out into the food. Instead, roast tomatoes yourself and blend them up for a delicious homemade soup.

Fertility-Reducing Food: French Fries

French fries are enjoyed around the globe. Even though they are just two simple ingredients, potatoes and oil, they are universally loved. Unfortunately, the mixture of starch and oil create chemicals as they are being fried that negatively impact health. One chemical in particular that has been shown to be detrimental in animal ovarian cells is called acrylamide. This chemical forms when certain types of foods, such as potatoes and grain products, are cooked at high temperatures, like deep-frying. The longer the cooking time, the higher content of acrylamide. It's a good thing to avoid starchy fried foods once you become pregnant also. A recent study found that when moms ate foods with high amounts of the chemical, their children were more likely to be overweight and obese later in life.

Organic fries won't make a difference, because the chemical still forms when organic potatoes are fried up. You are better off making your own healthier version of fries at home by baking sliced potatoes. And make sure you store your potatoes in a dark, cool place; this helps reduce the amount of this chemical from forming when they are prepared.

Fertility-Reducing Food: Foods Containing MSG

You've probably heard of MSG, which stands for monosodium glutamate. This chemical is added in order to enhance flavor, particularly in savory processed foods and Chinese food. It is also naturally found in foods like tomatoes and cheese, hydrolyzed vegetable protein, yeast extract, soy extracts, and protein isolate. Some people avoid it because they are sensitive to it (they may experience headaches, fatigue, and nausea, just to name a few adverse reactions) and if you're trying to get pregnant, it's a good idea for you to start avoiding foods that contain it as well. When tested in female rats, MSG has been shown to negatively impact the fallopian tubes and the oocytes, and in male mice it affects sperm cells. There is some debate about whether we need to completely avoid this additive due to its impact on fertility, but since it is in a majority of processed and fast foods, cutting out those foods will take a lot of the MSG out of your diet. Plus, as the name implies, monosodium glutamate is also a source of sodium, and too much salt isn't good for you, either. Nutrition labels must list if MSG has been added, so just make sure to read the ingredients of your favorite packaged foods and snacks so that you can start avoiding it.

Something to keep in mind: If a food naturally contains MSG (the ones noted above), then it does not need to be indicated on the label. The claims "No MSG" or "No added MSG" can't be used if the food contains it naturally, and MSG can't be hidden as "spices and flavoring" on the ingredients label.

Fertility-Reducing Food: Microwaved Buttered Popcorn

If you're in the mood for popcorn, it's better to make it the old-fashioned way and skip the microwavable bag. Yes, the bagged popcorn is already flavored, so it is easier, but those "flavors" are really just dressed-up chemicals that your body doesn't need. And read the nutrition label; it's full of everything you want to avoid. However, if you're not avoiding the bagged microwavable popcorn because of the high fat content, trans fat, inflammatory chemicals, or MSG, you should at least avoid it because of the bag that it comes in. The bag is lined with perfluorooctanoic acid (PFOA), which is another endocrine-disrupting chemical that impacts both male and female fertility, and it migrates into your food. Higher levels of these chemicals are associated with lower testosterone levels as well as abnormal changes to semen; in women it's associated with longer time to pregnancy (more on this chemical in chapter 8).

This doesn't mean that popcorn is off-limits, though. Popcorn is actually one of the healthier snacks to munch on, as it's naturally low in fat, a good source of fiber, and has polyphenols. Popping plain kernels in an electric popper is the best way to go. Doctor it up with whatever spices you want or try sprinkling on some nutritional yeast for a cheesy flavor without the extra saturated fat.

Fertility-Reducing Food: Swordfish

Although a diet higher in fish versus red meat is associated with better fertility outcomes, swordfish is one of the several types of fish that you want to avoid eating a lot of due to its high mercury content. Mercury has been shown to cause reproductive problems in both men and women, and causes damage to a baby's neurological development if the fetus is exposed to mercury in utero.

Unfortunately, cooking does not remove mercury, so choose your fish carefully. Salmon is almost always a great choice due to its excellent source of omega-3 fatty acids, but if you're tired of salmon, give Atlantic pollack a try. Pollack is a member of the cod family and is a white, flaky fish with a mild flavor. It really takes on the taste of the dish that it is prepared in, so it's a good fish to experiment with.

In general, if you're unsure if the fish you're about to eat is high in mercury, a good rule of thumb is to remember that larger fish are more likely to have higher levels of mercury (since they eat the smaller fish that ingest mercury when they eat plankton).

Highest mercury levels: tilefish, king mackerel, shark, swordfish, marlin, orange roughy, ahi tuna, bigeye tuna.

Lowest mercury levels: flounder, mahi mahi, vermilion snapper, tripletail, triggerfish, catfish, anchovies, perch.

Fertility-Reducing Food: Yellowtail Sushi Roll

Next time you order a sushi roll, make sure to avoid yellowtail. Like swordfish and sea bass, this fish contain high amounts of mercury, which are damaging to you and your partner's reproductive health. Overall, exposure to heavy metals, such as mercury, is negatively associated with ovarian health and overall pregnancy outcomes. You can still enjoy sushi, though! Just make a couple of easy changes. Swap yellowtail out for crab or eel, which are both lower in mercury. Crab is also an excellent source of vitamin B_{12}. Many places now have vegetarian rolls, which is another healthy choice to add to the list.

If you want to make your sushi even better, ask them to prepare your roll with brown rice instead of white. Sushi rolls may not feel like you're eating a lot of rice at once, but did you know that each roll is typically equal to one full cup of rice? This rice is very starchy and provides virtually no fiber, so it digests quickly and causes your blood sugar to spike. By having your rolls made with brown rice, you'll be getting more fiber, which will slow digestion. Plus, brown rice is a good source of selenium. One study found that women who were infertile had a lower selenium-to-mercury ratio, suggesting a relationship between the two metals, with selenium being protective. It is true that brown rice has more arsenic in it than white rice, but you can mitigate that when making it at home by parboiling the rice in pre-boiled water for five minutes before draining and refilling the water, then cooking it on a lower heat to absorb all the water. This method has been shown to retain the micronutrients and lower arsenic levels.

Lastly, skip the soy sauce and add some wasabi for a good source of vitamin C instead.

Fertility-Reducing Food: Beef

Only 3 ounces of beef provides about 25 grams of protein and almost 40 percent of your zinc and selenium needs and is a good source of iron as well. Unfortunately, beef is also linked to poorer fertility outcomes. Your risk of infertility seems to increase as your intake of animal protein does, especially when it's from red meat. So if you're worried that your diet is lacking protein, don't worry, because there are plenty of ways to get protein in your diet. Legumes, nuts, and tofu all have protein and are significantly lower in total fat than red meat. Since more and more research is showing that natural soy as part of a healthy diet may actually increase your chances of a successful pregnancy, tofu is a great way to get protein and other minerals like calcium that your body needs. Plus, tofu takes on the flavor of whatever you cook it with, so try swapping in tofu for beef next time you make a stir-fry for dinner. Another high-protein option is seafood, and when both men and women have fish in place of meat, better pregnancy outcomes have been observed. You don't have to completely avoid red meat, but lowering the amount you eat each week is associated with greater chances of a successful pregnancy. Plus, decreased red meat intake is associated with better overall health, and once you're caring for a little one, being healthier makes it easier!

• •

What About Salt?

You may have noticed that many of the foods listed above have something in common: they contain a lot of salt. Believe it or not, one of our favorite condiments turns out to be not so great when it comes to fertility. We've already seen through the research that a high salt intake can adversely affect our health in other ways, such as raising your blood pressure and increasing your risk of cardiovascular disease. Fortunately, numerous studies have shown that just reducing your salt intake (or specifically sodium) can lower blood pressure.

Unfortunately, there is not much research (if any) focused on salt intake and fertility outcomes in humans, but we can draw hypotheses from the many studies that have been done on mice and rats. For example, a study that came out in 2015 found that a high salt intake inhibits ovarian follicle development. Another study on laboratory animals found that excessive sodium intake by the mother caused a 50 percent decrease in litter size, suggesting a clear impact on fertility. We can also see effects on fertility in male rats. A high sodium intake in male rats reduces sperm production and decreases testosterone.

In a typical Western diet, it is estimated that people consume anywhere from 8 to 12 grams of sodium a day, whereas the recommendation is 1.5–2 grams per day. More than 70 percent of the sodium we eat comes from processed foods, such as boxed or canned goods, frozen dinners, cheeses, breads, soups, sandwiches, cold cuts and cured meats, and restaurant foods (especially fast food).

So do you need to go salt-free? Not at all. In fact, many of the recipes listed in chapters 5 and 7 include salt. What you *do* need to be mindful about is the amount of salt you are using. Salt is meant to be a flavor enhancer, not to make food taste salty. And since many processed foods use salt as a preservative or to mask the taste of other not-so-tasty ingredients, just by cutting back on your intake of processed foods you will reduce your salt intake.

Hidden Salt

It's important to know what's in your food. Just because something doesn't taste salty, doesn't mean it isn't full of salt. For example, a fast food Mexican salad bowl with lettuce, chicken, black beans, guacamole, cheese, and dressing has around 1.9 g of sodium. That's on the high end of your daily recommended intake in just one meal.

◆ ◆ ◆

Now you know not only the foods you should try to incorporate into your diet to boost your fertility but also the ones you should avoid or limit because they can be detrimental to health and fertility. The next step is to figure out a realistic plan to help you and your partner incorporate more of these fertility-promoting foods into your diet. In the next chapter, we will go over some menu ideas and some tips on how to stick with your new eating habits.

CHAPTER 7

Implementing the Plan: A Guide for You and Your Partner

We have covered a lot of information so far, and hopefully you are starting to see how some small changes to your diet can have a positive impact on not only your fertility but also your health in general. In this chapter, I want to cover a few important things that will make implementing the plan a breeze.

In this chapter, I will cover the importance of meal planning, and offer some weekly menus that you can use to help you to boost your fertility. One thing that you will notice about the Four-Week Fertility-Boosting Plan is that not only does it contain suggested menus, it also includes some "food for thought" each day-- kernels of advice to consider, which will help you to think about your habits, stressors, and other psychological aspects of your eating that can have an impact on how you feel and ultimately on your food choices. Anyone can look at a list of foods and recipes and plan to follow them, but really sticking to that plan involves something beyond just a food list. You need to dig deeper and ask some important questions about how you feel. The majority of unhealthy eating can be linked back to stress and lack of planning. Stress can make us choose less-healthy options, or can lead us to be unprepared (like if you are stressed about a work deadline and you end up having to get take-out again for dinner because you didn't think ahead). Later in this chapter, I am going to talk about stress and how you can recognize it, deal with it, and minimize it, so that it doesn't have a negative effect on your diet.

Four-Week Fertility-Boosting Plan

In chapter 6, I offered a bunch of easy-to-prepare recipes. Now we will incorporate those meals into a menu that can help boost your fertility though the optimal combination of the right kinds of foods. At the end of this chapter, I will give you some more recipes for snacks, desserts, and drinks, so you will have many options to choose from.

The beauty of these meal plans is that they are flexible and interchangeable. So, for example, if you don't feel like having eggs for breakfast, you can swap in a different type of breakfast. But, I highly encourage you to try all of these items, even if you aren't a fan of some of the ingredients. The reasons are: (1) having variety in your diet is important to your overall health, (2) you might be missing out on some important fertility-boosting nutrients if you avoid certain foods that contain them, and (3) you might like these foods when you taste them prepared differently than you have in the past.

SAMPLE MENU, WEEK 1

MONDAY:

B: Savory Mushroom, Onion, Thyme Oats (page 82)

L: Spicy Tuna and Chickpea Salad Sandwich (page 96)

D: Eggplant and Orzo with Turmeric and Tomato Sauce (page 80)

S: No-Bake Nut-Free Granola Bites with Honey and Lavender (page 94)

Food for Thought: Typically, diets or meal plans marketed as a "detox" or "cleanse" are the opposite of what you need. They often include severly restricting calories or cutting out whole food groups. This meal plan is not a "detox" or "cleanse." A typical detox or cleanse will likely just do more damage in the long run. Instead, long-term healthy eating plans involve eating enough calories and having a balanced diet.

TUESDAY:

B: Protein-Packed Papaya and Raspberry Breakfast Smoothie (page 90)

L: Turkey-Prosciutto Club with Homemade Chickpea Spread (page 97)

D: Vegetarian "Meatballs" with Tomato Sauce (page 79)

S: Homemade Lemon Hummus with cucumber slices (page 74)

Food for Thought: Forming habits requires repetition (with or without a dopamine response). Sticking to something for just a few days isn't necessarily going to change anything. That's why this meal plan is at least four weeks. Cooking, meal prepping, and meal planning aren't things that happen overnight. They take practice to not only become routine, but also to become easy and effortless.

WEDNESDAY:

B: Overnight Protein-Powered Oats with Berries (page 63)

L: Grilled Chicken Salad Rolls with Peanut Sauce (page 104)

D: Asian-Spiced Pork Spare Ribs over Sautéed Spinach (page 88)

S: Fertility Tonic (page 152)

Food for Thought: At first, you may find yourself craving your usual snacks, desserts, or even comfort food meals. Things that we associate with a rewarding feeling or sensation can be harder to do without, especially when we've created habits around them. Instead of ignoring these cravings, try to find something healthier you can replace it with. So, if you are craving apple pie, try this simple recipe: cut up an apple into chunks and place it in a microwave-safe mug with ¼ teaspoon each of cinnamon and cornstarch, plus 1 teaspoon of water, and stir.

Microwave for 2 minutes. It isn't apple pie, but it has that cinnamon-y apple goodness that can satisfy your craving.

THURSDAY:

B: Cashew and Pomegranate Granola Cereal (page 81)

L: Mixed Green Salad with Fertility-Boosting Nutty-Basil Vinaigrette (page 76)

D: Salmon and Yukon Gold Potato Hash (page 102)

S: Fertility-Boosting Fruit and Cheese Plate (page 153)

Food for Thought: Increasing your intake of omega-3 fatty acids is linked to increased chances of getting pregnant, so fish like salmon are essential to your fertility meal plan. Try incorporating plenty of salmon (wild-caught), herring, sardines, walnuts, chia seeds, flaxseed or flaxseed oil, and even supplements to get all the essential omega-3s that you need. Diversifying your sources of omega-3s helps ensure that you won't be exposed to too many pollutants that can be found in fish, like mercury and PBAs.

FRIDAY:

B: Mediterranean Scramble (page 92)

L: Avocado "Pesto" and Pasta (page 67)

D: Grilled Sardine and Cashew Shrimp Stir-Fry (page 77)

S: Chocolate-Chip Cookie Dough Sandwiches (page 157)

Food for Thought: For many people, staying in on a Friday night likely means sitting in front of the TV and mindlessly snacking on food, especially those chocolate-chip cookie dough sandwiches you're making for dessert. In some cases, replacing a food doesn't do the trick (see Wednesday's tip). Sometimes it's better to find a behavior that can derail a bad habit. Instead of mindless eating on the couch, eat dessert at the dinner table with no distractions and really enjoy it. Once you're done, then you can watch TV.

SATURDAY:

B: Banana-Bran Pancakes (page 63)

S: Matcha Latte with Easy Biscotti (page 154)

L: Roasted Pepper and Parmesan Cauliflower Florets with Homemade Lemon Hummus (page 74)

D: Spicy Canned Salmon with Chickpea Salad Cups (page 103)

Food for Thought: Having to go to a social event that involves food—think birthday parties, weddings, picnics--can make sticking to a meal plan difficult. Whether you're out with your friends, at a work event, or celebrating the holidays with your loved ones, preparation and flexibility is key. It's okay to indulge, but we want to avoid going overboard. Eat lunch or a snack at home before, bring your own healthy dish to the party, or keep an eye on your portion sizes and go for the veggies first.

SUNDAY:

B: Macadamia-Nut "Ricotta" Toast with Honey Glaze (page 69)

L: Have brunch or lunch out today (or gobble up some leftovers from the past week). If dining out, include lots of greens, and be sure to ask for your dressing on the side.

D: Lamb and Sweet Potato Pie (page 72)

S: Dark chocolate and dried cranberries

Food for Thought: A "cheat day," as the media commonly calls it, is a day in which you can eat anything you want (typically Sunday) because you ate well the rest of the week. This type of behavior can be exciting and rewarding, as well as reinforce the rewarding feeling of eating these particular "cheat" foods. However, it is better for your health (and mood) in the long run to maintain your healthy routine every day, and instead have indulgent (yet appropriate) meals or snacks here and there throughout the week.

WEEK 2:

MONDAY:

B: Overnight Protein-Powered Oats (with ½ chopped apple instead of berries) (page 63)

L: Fertility-Friendly "Sushi" Bowl (page 70)

D: Cherry-Glazed Chicken Kebabs (page 105)

S: Fertility Tonic (page 152)

Food for Thought: You may have noticed there are plenty of carbohydrates in this meal plan. Some of you may be wondering why, considering so many people rave about the keto diet for weight loss and overall health. In reality, the keto diet puts you at risk of nutrient deficiencies due to cutting out large food groups and can be harmful to your efforts to conceive. I don't recommend following the keto diet when trying to get pregnant.

TUESDAY:

B: Egg and Avocado Breakfast Sandwich (page 66)

L: Mixed Green Salad with Fertility-Boosting Nutty-Basil Vinaigrette (page 76)

D: Grilled Chicken Salad Rolls with Peanut Sauce (page 104)

S: Homemade Lemon Hummus with baby carrots (page 74)

Food for Thought: If you're feeling stressed, try to figure out why and how you can relieve your stress without automatically seeking out food. Self-medicating with food can feel rewarding in the moment, but it won't actually solve the problem. If you don't figure out what's stressing you out or what to do about it, you'll continue to seek out food, and probably not the healthiest food, either.

WEDNESDAY:

B: Cashew and Pomegranate Granola Cereal (page 81)

L: Grilled Sardine and Cashew Shrimp Stir-Fry (page 77)

D: Eggplant and Orzo with Turmeric and Tomato Sauce (page 80)

Ds: Shortbread Squares (page 158)

Food for Thought: Stress can make us more likely to gain weight thanks to the changes it causes in our body chemistry. Finding healthy ways to relieve stress is essential, especially when the stressor isn't necessarily something you can get away from. Try doing yoga, practicing meditation, going for a walk, cleaning your house, exercising, or listening to some music.

THURSDAY:

B: Garlicky Spinach Omelet with Sweet Potato Mash (page 97)

S: Matcha Latte with Easy Biscotti (page 154)

L: Grilled Three-Cheese Tuna Melt with Chicken Noodle Soup (page 100)

D: Spicy Canned Salmon with Chickpea Salad Cups (page 103)

Food for Thought: You'll notice that this meal plan includes plenty of whole foods, with minimal processing. That's because highly processed foods are rich in added sugars and high in saturated fats that not only lead to weight gain, but can also lead to changes in the brain that are similar to what we see in substance abuse disorders. To put it simply, highly processed foods are addicting, and that's a habit that is extremely hard to break and is detrimental to your health.

FRIDAY:

B: Protein-Packed Papaya and Raspberry Breakfast Smoothie (page 90)

L: Eat out for lunch today. Dining out can be tricky because so much restaurant food is unhealthy and loaded with added sugar, salts and other things you want to avoid. When eating out I suggest opting for a salad with dressing on the side, and adding a protein like chicken or shrimp.

D: Chicken Curry and Lentil Soup with Toasted Ciabatta (page 98)

S: Fertility-Boosting Fruit and Cheese Plate (page 153)

Food for Thought: Are you finding your old habits and cravings extremely difficult to give up? Do you think you might be addicted to food? Breaking an addiction to foods starts with figuring out what your triggers are for eating that food. Is it a certain emotion? A time of day? A mindless activity like watching TV? Or is it because you always eat this food when you eat or drink something else like always having cake when you drink coffee)? (See chapter 4 for signs that you might have an addiction to food.)

SATURDAY:

B: Mediterranean Scramble (page 92)

L: Spicy Tuna and Chickpea Salad Sandwich (page 96)

D: Vegetarian "Meatballs" with Tomato Sauce (page 79)

S: Baby-Friendly "Prosecco" with Nut and Cheese Tapas (page 156)

Food for Thought: Take baby steps. Going "cold turkey" on your old habits may work for a select few people, but, for most people, it doesn't. In fact, completely restricting all of your favorite or habitual foods can leave you feeling exhausted, overwhelmed, and like a failure (in the event of a slipup). Following this meal plan exactly is great, but it is not necessary. Take baby steps toward your goals and "wean off" the foods that are doing you more harm than good.

SUNDAY:

B: Waffles with Honey-Sweetened Frozen Yogurt (page 155)

L: Roasted Pepper and Parmesan Cauliflower Florets with Homemade Lemon Hummus (page 74)

D: Asian-Spiced Pork Spare Ribs over Sautéed Spinach (page 88)

S: No-Bake Nut-Free Granola Bites with Honey and Lavender (page 94)

Food for Thought: Remember to manage your portion sizes. If you don't already portion your food, you'll want to start now, especially for the junk. Use small containers or sealable baggies to portion ahead of time, so you won't have to think about it when a craving comes (or overindulge because you didn't prepare).

WEEK 3:

MONDAY:

B: Morning Summer Smoothie (page 153)

L: Roasted Chicken with Garlicky Kidney Beans and Collards (page 92)

D: Eggplant and Orzo with Turmeric and Tomato Sauce (page 80)

S: Chocolate-Chip Cookie Dough Sandwiches (page 157)

Food for Thought: Keeping plenty of fresh, healthy food in your house isn't enough; it needs to be ready to eat. Just having a head of broccoli in your refrigerator isn't going to help. Buy precut veggies or wash and chop them once you get home from the grocery store. Junk food is typically "easy" food, which makes us so much more likely to grab a bag of chips or pour a soda.

TUESDAY:

B: Avocado toast with hard-boiled egg

L: Use leftovers from the past few days as lunch today.

D: Lamb and Sweet Potato Pie (page 72)

S: Baby-Friendly "Prosecco" with Nut and Cheese Tapas (page 156)

Food for Thought: If you're not ready to remove the junk from your house, the next best thing is to put it away and out of sight. Even better, put it up on a very high shelf, making it more difficult to access. Often, we don't crave something unless we see it or smell it, so put that junk food away!

WEDNESDAY:

B: Banana-Bran Pancakes (page 63)

L: Grilled Three-Cheese Tuna Melt with Chicken Noodle Soup (page 100)

D: Date night! Order in your favorite dish from your favorite place. You have been doing so well with eating healthy, so treat yourself to what you enjoy the most!

S: Fertility Tonic (page 152)

Food for Thought: Have you been sleeping well lately? Eating healthy is not just about the food. Getting a good night's sleep is essential to feeling your best and making good choices. Food cravings tend to increase when you're sleepy, so make sure to take some time this week to focus on good sleep hygiene.

THURSDAY:

B: Greek yogurt, blueberries, cashews, and honey

L: Kale, roasted chickpeas, roasted butternut squash, avocado, and egg/tofu warm salad

D: Salmon and Yukon Gold Potato Hash (page 102)

S: Banana Bread with Almond Frosting (page 158)

Food for Thought: Remember in chapter 4 how we talked about routine stress? How all of those little things in our day can add up and cause chronic stress on our bodies? Take ten minutes today to think about ways in which you can reduce or eliminate at least one or two of these stressors. Reducing your stress will help you eat, sleep, and feel better.

FRIDAY:

B: Overnight Protein-Powered Oats with Fruit (page 63)

L: Turkey-Prosciutto Club with Homemade Chickpea Spread (page 97)

D: Chicken Curry and Lentil Soup with Toasted Ciabatta (page 98)

S: Grapes and pistachio mix

Food for Thought: Trying to accomplish anything is at least a little bit easier, if not a whole lot easier, if we have someone else supporting us, whether they're cheering us on or joining us in the journey. When it comes to fertility, getting your partner involved in some way is essential, considering that the health of both partners is key to conceiving.

SATURDAY:

B: Macadamia-Nut "Ricotta" Toast with Honey Glaze (page 69)

L: Fertility-Friendly "Sushi" Bowl (page 70)

D: Lamb and Sweet Potato Pie (page 72)

S: Fertility-Boosting Fruit and Cheese Plate (page 153)

Food for Thought: Although this meal plan is full of animal sources like chicken, turkey, lamb, and fish, that doesn't mean you can't follow a vegetarian or vegan diet if you want to conceive. However, it's important to look back to chapter 3 and brush up on ways to increase your nutrient intake if you are vegetarian or vegan, as certain vitamins and minerals may be lacking, depending on what and how you eat.

SUNDAY:

B: Think outside the traditional breakfast box! Peel and cube a sweet potato, then boil it for about 25 minutes. Mash it and add walnuts, raisins, and cinnamon (optional side of egg). It's a delicious and healthy way to start your day.

L: Tuna avocado salad with whole-grain crackers, cheese, and cucumbers

D: Buffalo Cauliflower "Wings" with Avocado Aioli Dipping Sauce Pie (page 84)

S: No-Bake Nut-Free Granola Bites with Honey and Lavender (page 94)

Food for Thought: It's not always easy to stay motivated when it's impossible to know when you'll actually get pregnant. Will it be this month? Will it be next year? When this happens, it's important to remind yourself why you're trying to change your habits. Write down what you'll gain from these changes to keep your motivation up.

WEEK 4:

MONDAY:

B: Greek yogurt, blueberries, cashews, and honey

L: Easy Turmeric Turkey, Sweet Potato, and Zucchini Bowl (page 73)

D: Chicken Curry and Lentil Soup with Toasted Ciabatta (page 98)

S: Homemade Lemon Hummus with whole-grain crackers (page 74)

Food for Thought: This week, whenever you have a food craving, I want you to ask yourself, "Am I really hungry?" Learning to differentiate between your internal hunger cues and other cues like emotions will help you make better decisions when it comes to food.

TUESDAY:

B: Power green smoothie: avocado, banana, date, spinach, almond milk

L: Grilled Chicken Salad Rolls with Peanut Sauce (page 104)

D: Leftover night! Clear out the refrigerator and eat up what you have left over from the past few days.

S: No-Bake Nut-Free Granola Bites with Honey and Lavender (page 94)

Food for Thought: Week 4 may seem like the home stretch, but changing your habits doesn't just stop after four weeks. This is not meant to be a one-time diet plan that changes your life in four weeks. Instead, it's a starting point to help you create new habits and routines that you can continue to work on after you get through this last week.

WEDNESDAY:

B: Egg and Avocado Breakfast Sandwich (page 66)

L: Use some leftovers from the past few days for lunch today.

D: Cherry-Glazed Chicken Kebabs (page 105)

S: Sliced apple with sunflower seed butter and cinnamon

Food for Thought: Meal prepping doesn't mean you have to prepare every single meal that you're going to eat for the week on a Sunday. That's definitely helpful, if you want to avoid cooking at all costs during the week, but it doesn't have to be that way. Another version of meal prepping that's helpful and still saves time is batch cooking. Cook several ingredients that can be made in large batches and saved in the refrigerator to eat throughout the week, like roasted veggies, grains, legumes, etc. Chop and prep other fresh ingredients like raw veggies or greens. By doing some simple prep work, when you need to put together a meal, all you have to do is pick and choose which ingredients you want that day and throw everything in a dish or container and enjoy!

THURSDAY:

B: Morning Summer Smoothie (page 153)

L: Grilled Three-Cheese Tuna Melt with Chicken Noodle Soup (page 100)

D: Buffalo Cauliflower "Wings" with Avocado Aioli Dipping Sauce (page 84)

S: Homemade Lemon Hummus with baby carrots (page 74)

Food for Thought: If you're not someone who spends all day at home or has constant access to a kitchen, it's important to be prepared by having snacks on hand that you can take anywhere. They may not be a part of this meal plan, but having snacks like low-sugar energy bars, trail mixes, or other shelf-stable snacks like crunchy chickpeas can be a lifesaver and keep you from overeating at your next meal due to being overly hungry.

FRIDAY:

B: Garlicky Spinach Omelet with Sweet Potato Mash (page 87)

L: Kale, roasted chickpeas, roasted butternut squash, avocado, and egg/tofu warm salad

D: Eggplant and Orzo with Turmeric and Tomato Sauce (page 80)

S: Grapes and pistachio mix

Food for Thought: Take a moment to reflect on the support you've had so far in this process. Is there anything you would want to change? Do you need more or less support? Consider what you need and if you need to renegotiate how you receive support with your partner, friend, or whoever is in this with you.

SATURDAY:

B: Savory Mushroom, Onion, Thyme Oats (page 82)

L: Spicy Tuna and Chickpea Salad Sandwich (page 96)

D: Chicken Curry and Lentil Soup with Toasted Ciabatta (page 98)

S: Chocolate-Chip Cookie Dough Sandwiches (page 157)

Food for Thought: Now that you're about to embark on your own meal plan, take ten minutes today to think about the meals you liked and didn't like from this meal plan. Think about the cooking methods you found delicious and easy versus the ones you probably won't do much again. Then, plan out some meals you can make on your own in the coming week and create a grocery list. Also, it's definitely okay to eat the same thing every day for breakfast, or lunch, or dinner. A balance of variety and routine is the key to success.

SUNDAY:

B: Avocado toast with smoked salmon

S: Trail mix: goji berries, chopped dates, almonds, pistachios, sunflower seeds

L: Caprese avocado salad: mixed greens, avocado, tomato, mozzarella, roasted chicken, basil, balsamic vinegar

D: Asian-Spiced Pork Spare Ribs over Sautéed Spinach (page 88)

Food for Thought: When working toward our goals, it's important to do a self-evaluation every once in a while. What was week 1 like for you versus week 4? Have you noticed any changes in how you feel, the choices you're making, or your cravings? Use this self-evaluation to figure out what you need to do next and how you can keep making progress toward your goals.

The Importance of Meal Planning

I can't stress enough how important it is to plan out your meals. Not only does planning out what you will eat help you to ensure you are eating a healthy diet, but it also reduces stress and poor decision making. Planning out your meals doesn't mean that you have to cancel all of your last-minute dinner invitations. Meal planning involves planning what you will make at home and also planning what you will eat when you are out. If you are headed to a restaurant, check out the menu online before you arrive so you can look over your options and not have to make a rushed decision.

Stress and Your Fertility

We've talked about stress a lot so far, but what exactly is stress? Stress is any threat, like a threat to our homeostasis or well-being, either physical or psychological. Stress has clear effects on our mood and behavior, both in the short term and in the long run. Stress can be good, such as the stress that drives you to study for an important exam or finish a big project on time. Stress can be physical, such as the stress of working out our bodies, which eventually can help shape us into athletes.

On the other hand, not-so-great stress can be detrimental to you both physically and emotionally. If you have a stressful job, you're probably feeling stressed on a daily basis. Over time, this constant stress can wreak havoc on your body. You may start getting sick more often, craving sweets or comfort foods all the time, or even have trouble remembering things. Stress could even make it easier to gain weight, and harder to lose it.

This is not unlike the stress that you may experience when trying to get pregnant. There's no question that there is some sort of relationship between stress and your fertility. Studies in women, both in general populations and infertile women, show that stress is associated with decreased conception rates, longer menstrual cycles, and lower success rates in assisted reproduction treatments; in some women, chronic stress may diminish the ovarian reserve. Clearly, stress can impede your ability to get pregnant. So, how do we reduce stress and avoid stress in the future?

Obviously, using food to eat away your stress is not the answer—especially since the food we typically turn to in stressful times are not the healthiest: sugar-filled cakes and candies; fat-laden, comforting carbs; super-salty, fried snacks. But there is one way to reduce stress with food. You could start meal planning. In many cases, being prepared is a surefire way to avoid stress eating the unhealthy food. And cooking in itself could be a great way to relax, since it forces you to focus on the task at hand and get your mind off of the things that are bothering you.

In addition to eating well, it's important to engage in other stress-reducing activities. Some of the best ways to reduce stress include getting plenty of exercise, reducing your caffeine and alcohol intake (improving your sleep is key), spending time with friends and family (the ones who don't stress you out!), spending time with your pet if you have one, taking a yoga or meditation class, and learning to say "no."

Speaking about learning to say "no" . . . This can do wonders for your stress. Trying to attend every social event, taking on every project at work, helping every single one of your friends when they need a favor, and trying to have a baby on top of it all can be absolutely exhausting. It's okay to set some limits for yourself and just take time to relax whenever you can.

• •

"Just try not to stress . . ."

If one more person had said that to me when I was trying to get pregnant, I would have screamed. Although I am sure the people who made this comment meant no harm, I took it as an insult. Every time I heard this I thought "Do you really think I would be stressed *on purpose* knowing that it isn't good for a pregnancy or health in general?" No one is *trying* to be stressed, but when you are desperately wanting to have a baby, and you are trying to balance your life, relationships, career, and other things, on top of the added angst that can come along with having a hard time conceiving, who *wouldn't* be stressed? It is completely normal to feel anxious about trying to get pregnant, but you do want to keep it in check so that it won't hurt your health or hinder your chances of conceiving. Try finding a healthy outlet for your stress, like working out in the morning, or using a meditation app.

• •

◆ ◆ ◆

Getting Your Partner Onboard

Having a support system, whether that be your partner, a friend, coworker, or even a health professional, can greatly increase your chances of trying to change your eating habits and sticking with these changes. There is a lot of research today that shows how impactful social support can be when embarking on some sort of lifestyle change or weight-loss program. It's kind of a no-brainer. When you have your partner onboard, the journey can become much easier, more motivating, and more fun. Think about it this way: A marathon runner may be the only one actually running the race, but without the support of a coach, or her family and friends cheering her on, it would be that much harder to cross the finish line.

When it comes to fertility, having your partner onboard is even more important considering that male fertility shouldn't be left out of the equation. If both partners are involved in making lifestyle changes, you are that much more likely to get pregnant and have a healthy baby. Even if your partner isn't involved in the biological part of the process (i.e., same-sex couples), having your partner onboard is key to maintaining a peaceful home environment and for motivation and accountability.

If you don't have a support system, the good news is that getting support can be pretty easy these days. For example, if you don't have a close social circle, you can typically find support groups within your community or even online. Even if you do have a partner, family, or close friend to turn to, support sometimes doesn't come easy and you may even find that some people actually discourage you on your journey.

Let's say you are going to change your eating habits in order to lose some weight and improve your fertility. You may hear things like "You don't need to lose weight" or "Don't be silly, that won't do anything," or it may be that your partner resents you for spending more time in the gym, for example. There are so many ways in which people can be unsupportive, just as there are many explanations as to why someone might not be supportive of you. People may have insecurities of their own, or they may not understand the science or purpose behind these changes. This doesn't mean the person doesn't care about you or your well-being. Sometimes it just takes a little extra effort on your end to explain why you want to make these lifestyle changes in order to help your partner or friend understand. Typically, explaining why it's important to you is enough to get the support you need.

Although it's rare, some people (although rarely) still may not be willing to give support, in which case it would be best to not discuss what you are doing with them and instead focus on other topics. At the end of the day, the best thing you can do is seek support from those who are positive contributors to your life and willing to give you encouragement.

Understanding What You Are Eating

Another barrier that can get in the way of eating healthy is not know-ing which foods are actually healthy! Information is key, but some-times the information that we are given isn't so easy to understand. Take the Nutrition Facts label. These labels contain a lot of informa-tion, but do you know what to look for to determine whether or not something is a healthy food choice? Let's go over some tips to help make these labels easier to decipher:

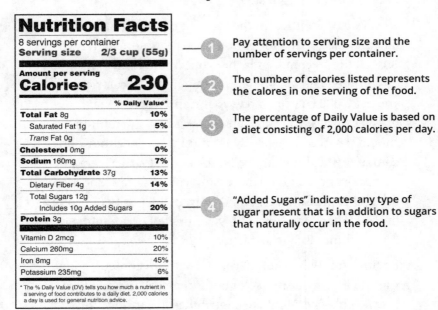

Nutrition Facts

8 servings per container
Serving size   2/3 cup (55g)

Amount per serving
Calories   230

	% Daily Value*
Total Fat 8g	**10%**
Saturated Fat 1g	**5%**
Trans Fat 0g	
Cholesterol 0mg	**0%**
Sodium 160mg	**7%**
Total Carbohydrate 37g	**13%**
Dietary Fiber 4g	**14%**
Total Sugars 12g	
Includes 10g Added Sugars	**20%**
Protein 3g	
Vitamin D 2mcg	10%
Calcium 260mg	20%
Iron 8mg	45%
Potassium 235mg	6%

* The % Daily Value (DV) tells you how much a nutrient in a serving of food contributes to a daily diet. 2,000 calories a day is used for general nutrition advice.

1. Pay attention to serving size and the number of servings per container.

2. The number of calories listed represents the calores in one serving of the food.

3. The percentage of Daily Value is based on a diet consisting of 2,000 calories per day.

4. "Added Sugars" indicates any type of sugar present that is in addition to sugars that naturally occur in the food.

1. Every Nutrition Facts label provides information about the contents of exactly one serving of that food, which is defined in the first line, right below the title "Nutrition Facts." This is important to keep in mind when reading a nutrition label because you might be consuming more than one serving. For instance, some beverages list the energy and nutrient information for a single serving of that drink, however, the nutrition label may also indicate that there are 1.5 or 2 servings per bottle or container. Therefore, if you plan to drink the entire bottle, you should multiply the values listed on the label by 1.5 or 2 in order to see how much you are really consuming.

2. The second piece of information listed on a nutrition label is the number of calories *per serving*.

3. Next, the label provides a breakdown of the nutrients in the food, indicated as both the actual amount of a nutrient present in one serving (on the left side) and as a percentage of the daily recommended intake (percent Daily Value) of that nutrient (on the right side).

4. Always pay attention to the amount of saturated and trans fat contained in the foods you eat. The American Heart Association recommends that you should limit your intake of saturated fats to 5–6 percent of your daily calories. So if you eat 2,000 calories a day, that translates to a maximum of 120 calories from saturated fat per day. In addition, you should try to completely avoid trans fats, since they don't confer any health benefits; on the contrary, they can only damage your health by increasing your risk for cancer and other chronic illnesses. Thankfully, the majority of products in the United States have now eliminated or are in the process of eliminating trans fats.

5. Be mindful of the cholesterol and sodium content, as you want to limit your intake of both to maintain good health (excess cholesterol intake contributes to cardiovascular disease and excess sodium leads to high blood pressure).

6. The next piece of information is the carbohydrate content of the food. This includes total carbohydrate, dietary fiber, and sugar content per serving. It is a good idea to choose foods with more fiber and less sugars to help you achieve the recommended daily intake of fiber and limit the calories from added sugars, which, if consumed in excess, may lead to weight gain.

7. The last macronutrient listed on the label is protein. According to the National Research Council, women between the ages of 19 and 70 should consume approximately 46 grams of protein per day, but that amount can vary based on activity levels (less is needed if you are inactive, more if you are very active). In general, protein intake in adult women should be 10–35 percent of all calories.

8. Listed next are the four vitamins and minerals that are required to be reported on each food package: vitamins A and C, calcium, and iron. These are expressed as percentages of the daily recommended intake. However, it is important to keep in mind that all values in a Nutrition Facts label are based on a diet consisting of 2,000 calories per day (which is the amount of calories that an *average* person needs each day). If your daily energy goal is higher or lower than 2,000 kcal, your needs for the nutrients will also differ accordingly. With that said, this label is still a helpful guide to help you better understand what the nutrient density of that food is. Remember, nutrient-dense foods are those that deliver the most beneficial nutrients with relatively few calories (e.g., a cup of kale is more nutrient dense than a cupcake). Also, toward the bottom of the label, there is a small table comparing the percent Daily Values of a 2,000 kcal/day and a 2,500 kcal/day diet, indicating the different amounts for some nutrients. Note that the percent Daily Values for cholesterol and sodium do not vary with different caloric intakes as 300 mg of cholesterol and 2.4 grams of sodium are the upper limits of the daily recommended amounts (although less

sodium should be consumed in certain conditions such as high blood pressure).

9. The last part of the label indicates the number of calories per gram of each macronutrient: carbohydrate and protein each have 4 calories per gram, while fat has 9 calories per gram.

10. While you don't have to read the list of ingredients included at the bottom of a nutrition label each time you buy the same food (although ingredients do change from time to time in the same food product, often without an indication, especially when it comes to food additives or an increase in the sugar or fat content), it is a good habit when considering between products to determine which is the healthiest option. Some nutritionists say that you should avoid foods that have more than five ingredients. While this can be very true for certain foods that contain additives, emulsifiers, food dyes, preservatives, thickening agents, flavor enhancers, added sugars and fats, more does not necessarily mean worse when it comes to less-processed or whole foods, such as trail mix (some contain ten or more ingredients, all of which are perfectly healthy). So when examining a list of ingredients, look for words that aren't familiar or that make you wonder, "why does this need to be in here?" Unfortunately, food manufacturers are often quite clever when it comes to hiding the "bad stuff" with terms that you may either not understand or that might sound healthy, which brings me to my next point . . .

Know Your Enemy

Food manufacturers use all sorts of lingo to disguise ingredients that they know you know are not great for you. If a food contains sugar, for example, the label won't always list the word "sugar" as an ingredient. Instead, there are a plethora of code words that can be put on the label instead, and while those ingredients might have been made in different ways, essentially, they are sugar. Take a look at page 112, which lists some examples of names for added sugars that you may find in the ingredients list of a food label. Brown sugar may sound like a healthier alternative to white granulated sugar, but its effects on your body are no different, and it has the same nutritional value (or lack thereof) as regular white table sugar. Similarly, solid fats can be listed under a variety of names. While "coconut oil" sounds much healthier than "pork fat," they are both saturated fats that have similar effects on your health. When it comes to ingredients like sugars and fats, which we are recommended to consume in limited amounts, moderation is key. While the occasional bite won't kill you, try your best to avoid foods with added sugars, saturated fats, large amounts of sodium, and ingredients you can't pronounce.

Aim for Optimal Nutrient Proportions and Dietary Variety

You should aim to consume the recommended proportions of all three macronutrients, which for adults who are nineteen years old and older means that 45–65 percent of all daily calories should come from carbohydrates, 10–35 percent from protein, and 20–35 percent from fat. In addition, you should aim for variety in your diet instead of eating the same foods over and over again. Consuming many different foods will not only help you increase the chances of getting all the nutrients you need but will also reduce the risk of consuming too much of what your body does not need, such as mercury in fish (if you regularly eat the same kind of fish and it's high in mercury).

• •

Are All Proteins the Same?

Most people usually have no trouble meeting the daily protein requirement, as protein is found in many different sources and diets deficient in protein are now quite rare. However, not all proteins are created equal, and are "ranked" by their biological value, which reflects how well the protein you consume gets integrated into your body. Protein sources that have the highest biological value include milk, soybeans and soybean milk, eggs, cheese, rice, quinoa, beef, and fish. Another method used to evaluate protein is Protein Digestibility Corrected Amino Acid Score (PDCAAS), which indicates how well your body can digest the protein. Foods with high rankings on the PDCAAS scale include milk, egg whites, soybeans, beef, chickpeas, black beans, fruits, vegetables, and legumes. As you can see, there is quite a bit of overlap between the two, making it easier for you to choose foods that are both high in their biological value as well as readily digestible.

• •

However, another factor to consider is if you are consuming *complete* or high-quality protein. *Complete protein* sources are foods that contain all the essential amino acids (amino acids are the building blocks of protein) in "perfect" proportions—in amounts that are most optimal for your body to support its functions. The nine essential amino acids are called "essential" because you need to get them from your diet because your body cannot make them (as opposed to the nonessential amino acids). The majority of animal foods have complete protein (for example, eggs, milk, cheese, fish, poultry, meat), whereas plant foods (such as nuts, seeds, grains, beans) tend to lack one or more amino acids. Does that mean that you should only focus on animal foods? No. You can get all the protein you need by eating plant foods alone *if* you eat a variety of them. While they are considered incomplete because they lack one or more of the essential amino acids, combining complementary proteins (two or more protein sources that together contain all the essential amino acids, such as brown rice and beans) can provide you with all the essential amino acids. Further, complementary proteins don't need to be eaten within the same meal; you will absorb everything just fine if you eat them within the same day. Ideally, however, you should try to get a balanced mix of both animal and plant proteins, because in addition to the protein, you're also getting vitamins and minerals from them.

It's the Big Picture That Matters

While all the little things certainly count, like what snacks you eat in the afternoon on any given day, it's the overall pattern that matters most. The foods you regularly choose, the average amount of nutrients you get in the span of 2–3 days, the number of alcoholic beverages you drink and the frequency with which you drink them, the volume of water that you drink, and the amount of fiber you consume with your foods is what makes up your regular dietary pattern. If your *overall* dietary pattern is healthy, then a small piece of cake, ice cream, or candy bar every once in a blue moon won't make much of a difference and won't lead to weight gain or obesity. With that said, dessert and junk foods should remain as only occasional treats, and not regularly eaten items.

Hydration

Essential in every stage of life, drinking plenty of water and keeping yourself hydrated is especially important for a healthy diet. Drinking water requires little time but may take a little bit of planning. Make sure you always have a glass or bottle of water around. Try not to wait until you actually feel the sensation of thirst (at that point, your body is already about 2 percent dehydrated) and drink frequently throughout the day. This will not only keep you properly hydrated but also ensure that you feel well (dehydration can cause headaches, cramps, and constipation).

• •

Healthful Hint

If you are wondering if maybe you are pregnant but it's too early to tell, should you ramp up your calorie intake just in case you are eating for two? Nope! This might be shocking and contrary to what your mother, friends and others have told you, but you actually don't need *any* extra calories in the first trimester of pregnancy. It is important, however, to be sure that you are getting the appropriate amount of calories based on your BMI, age, and activity level. For example, if you are 31–50 years old and have a BMI of 21.5 (within the normal range), you need about 1,800–2,400 calories per day depending on your level of physical activity. If you are interested in finding out how many calories that you specifically may need each day, you can enter your age, weight, height, sex, and physical activity information into several calorie calculators available online.

• •

Additional Recipes: Snacks, Desserts and Beverages

In addition to the recipes for breakfast, lunch, and dinner in chapter 5, here are some additional snack and beverage ideas to help fill in gaps when you need them.

Fertility Tonic

This nutrient-dense drink is a great way to start your morning and also boosts your fertility. This tonic is loaded with antioxidants, and the orange provides you with a healthy dose of vitamin C, to boot!

Makes 1 serving.

1	peeled orange (or ⅓ cup fortified orange juice)
1	small carrot (raw or cooked), peeled and roughly chopped
½	small beet (raw or cooked), roughly chopped
1 teaspoon	grated fresh ginger
6 fluid ounces	maple water (or coconut water)

Blend ingredients together until smooth. Add ice as desired to the blender. Drink immediately.

Morning Summer Smoothie

This smoothie is a good way to get nutritious calories, and it's full of electrolytes to keep you feeling your best. This recipe is packed with folate, potassium, sodium, and calcium, among many other important fertility-promoting micronutrients. Surprisingly, although avocados are particularly famous for their unsaturated fat content, they're also a great source of folate (59 micrograms in ½ avocado), which is needed before pregnancy. Lastly, the fat from the coconut and avocado will help to counterbalance the sugar from the banana, and keep you feeling full longer.

Makes 1 serving.

½	avocado
1	frozen banana
2½ tablespoons	unsweetened shredded coconut
1 cup	unsweetened almond milk
pinch	sea salt

Blend ingredients together in a blender. Add more or less almond milk until desired consistency is reached.

Fertility-Boosting Fruit and Cheese Plate

Blackberries are arguably one of the healthiest fruits you can eat. Berries have a low glycemic index compared to other fruits due to their high fiber content. One cup is only about 60 calories and provides your body with essential nutrients like potassium, magnesium, and anti-inflammatory compounds. Plus, the rich flavor of blackberries pairs really well with soft goat cheese.

Makes 1 serving.

1 cup	organic blackberries (or raspberries)
1 slice	whole-grain seeded bread
1 ounce	reduced-fat goat cheese
1 teaspoon	honey

Wash the berries under cold running water, set aside and pat dry.

Toast bread, and, while it's still warm, smear goat cheese on toast to make it slightly melted. Lightly drizzle honey across the bread and cheese. Cut bread into four pieces and top with half of the berries or enjoy the berries separately.

Matcha Latte with Easy Biscotti

Matcha is powdered green tea. It contains many different antioxidants and is also a good source of the amino acid theanine, which has been shown to help with reducing stress. Purchasing a matcha latte at your local café can cost over $5, so making it yourself is a good way to save money and still enjoy the health benefits. The biscotti only contain five ingredients, are easy to make, and have no sugar!

Makes 3–4 biscotti and 1 latte.

FOR THE BISCOTTI
¼ cup	almonds
¼ cup	pistachio nuts
1 teaspoon	almond or vanilla extract
¼ cup	liquid egg whites

FOR THE LATTE
1 cup	unsweetened almond milk
1 teaspoon	honey
1 tablespoon	matcha powder

Preheat oven to 275° F. Pulse nuts in a blender until they have a flour-like consistency while still keeping some chunks. Remove from the blender and add extract of your choice and liquid egg whites. Stir until all ingredients are blended. Roll out 3–4 "cookies" on parchment paper. Bake for 10–12 minutes. While biscotti are baking, boil the unsweetened almond milk, and whisk in the matcha powder until smooth. Sweeten with honey. Serve latte alongside biscotti.

Waffles with Honey-Sweetened Frozen Yogurt

Waffles are a really easy way to make sure that you're not skipping breakfast. This recipe is great because unlike many of the store-bought frozen varieties, this one doesn't contain three different types of sugar or inflammatory oils. This homemade sweetened frozen yogurt is also a good source of calcium and protein. This recipe doubles as a dessert!

Makes 2–3 servings.

FOR THE FROZEN YOGURT

¾ cup	nonfat Greek yogurt
splash	almond milk (to help blend)
1	frozen large chopped banana

FOR THE WAFFLES

½ cup	almond or coconut flour
1 cup	whole wheat flour
1 teaspoon	baking soda
1 teaspoon	cinnamon
½ teaspoon	salt
1 cup	unsweetened almond milk
2	large eggs
1 teaspoon	vanilla extract
1 teaspoon	honey
	cooking spray

To prepare the frozen yogurt, add yogurt, almond milk, and frozen banana to a blender and mix until smooth. Transfer to a bowl and place in freezer for at least 1 hour. To prepare the waffles, sift together flours, baking soda, cinnamon, and salt. In a separate bowl, mix almond milk, eggs, vanilla, and honey. Add wet ingredients to the dry, and whisk until well combined.

Spray waffle iron with cooking spray, pour batter onto hot iron, and cook until browned. Top with frozen yogurt and enjoy!

Baby-Friendly Prosecco with Nut and Cheese Tapas

Although the research on the intake of alcohol and fertility is still inconclusive, avoiding it to be on the safe side is probably a good idea. That's not a problem, as there are now plenty of varieties of "alcohol-free" or "mocktail" versions of your favorite wines and bubbly beverages. But it's more fun to make it yourself so you can doctor it up however you would like. Staying hydrated (without alcohol) is important, so drink up while enjoying a healthy dose of anti-inflammatory fats from a handful of nuts and a sharp taste of cheese to get some added calcium and protein. This snack is not only tasty but also an excellent balance of macronutrients to keep you full.

Makes 1 serving.

1 tablespoon	sugar
1 tablespoon	water
½	grapefruit
8–12 ounces	grapefruit-flavored sparkling water
	basil or mint for garnish
¼ cup	mixed nuts (try including Brazil nuts)
1 ounce	sharp cheddar, cut into small pieces

Bring sugar and water to a boil in a small saucepan. Boil until the sugar dissolves, stirring constantly. Allow the mixture to cool. Cut 1–2 thin slices of grapefruit from the half and set aside from the rest. Pour the grapefruit-flavored sparkling water into any fancy glass, add in the sugar/water mixture, and squeeze the unsliced grapefruit. Mix together and add the mint or basil (your choice) and 2 thin slices of grapefruit for garnish. Arrange nuts and cheese on the plate and serve along with the beverage.

Chocolate-Chip Cookie Dough Sandwiches

Instead of using ice cream or frosting as the middle to your sandwiches, this recipe calls for bananas. Frozen bananas that have been sliced prior to freezing whip up to a consistency (and sweetness) similar to ice cream, but with none of the fat or added chemicals. Not to worry, these cookie dough sandwiches don't contain eggs, so you can lick the spoon with no fear. Plus, the dark chocolate provides you with lots of antioxidants, making it a guilt-free snack!

Makes about 2 sandwiches.

3 tablespoons	smooth peanut butter
1½ teaspoons	vanilla extract, divided
5	dates
½ cup	almond meal
½ cup	oatmeal
1–2 tablespoons	water (if needed)
¼ cup + 1 tablespoon	dark chocolate chips
2	presliced frozen bananas*

Combine peanut butter, 1 teaspoon vanilla, dates, almond meal and oatmeal in a food processor. Blend until smooth. If the mixture is too dry or thick add a little water and process again. Remove mixture from food processor, and fold in ¼ cup of the chocolate chips. Divide the dough into four balls, flatten slightly with a spatula, and refrigerate for about 30 minutes. While the cookies are chilling, make the "ice cream." Using a blender, blend the bananas* and ½ teaspoon vanilla until smooth, sprinkle in 1 tablespoon of chocolate chips. Once the cookies are chilled, spoon the banana "ice cream" onto two cookies, then top them off with the remaining cookies. Serve immediately.

---

* If you wanted to lower the amount of natural sugar from the banana ice cream, you can substitute one zucchini (peeled, sliced and then frozen) for one of the bananas.

Shortbread Squares

Typically shortbread is not a food that is associated with being healthy. Although it's traditionally made with few ingredients, these ingredients are mainly sugar and fat, which isn't a great combo for reproductive health. Not to worry, as this version is lower in saturated fat, and since it's made with whole wheat flour and chickpea flour instead of bleached white flour, there is the added bonus of fiber and protein!

Makes about 10 cookies.

1 teaspoon	vanilla extract
⅓ cup	honey
2 tablespoons	melted coconut oil
1 cup	whole wheat flour
¾ cup	chickpea flour
¼ teaspoon	baking soda

Preheat oven to 325° F. Line a sheet pan with parchment paper. In a medium-size bowl, mix the vanilla extract, honey, and coconut oil together with a hand mixer until well blended. Add in the whole wheat flour, chickpea flour, and baking soda and mix until completely blended. Remove the dough and press it down evenly into the sheet pan. Bake for 20–25 minutes, until golden. Once cooled, cut into squares. Store in an airtight container for up to five days.

Banana Bread with Almond Frosting

This recipe uses anti-inflammatory olive oil instead of vegetable oils that are more commonly used in baking, as well as Greek yogurt to keep it lower in calories while upping the protein. Since avoiding sweets that are high in sugar is important when trying to get pregnant (and in general), using ripe bananas instead of sugar not only adds at least 2 grams of fiber per serving, but also adds over 1500 mg of potassium to your diet, which is important for both male and female reproductive health.

Makes 5–6 servings.

FOR THE BANANA BREAD

1 cup	whole wheat flour
¾ cup	almond flour
1 teaspoon	cinnamon
½ teaspoon	nutmeg
1 teaspoon	baking soda
1	egg
and 1	egg white
¼ cup	olive oil
¼ cup	nonfat Greek yogurt
¼ cup	honey
3–4	mashed ripe bananas

FOR THE ALMOND FROSTING

½ cup	whipped fat-free cream cheese
¼ cup	confectioners' sugar
1 teaspoon	almond extract
¼ cup	finely chopped almonds

Preheat oven to 350° F. Spray loaf pan with nonstick olive oil cooking spray. Mix the flours, cinnamon, nutmeg, and baking soda together in a medium-sized bowl. In a separate bowl, mix together the eggs, olive oil, Greek yogurt, honey, and mashed banana. Combine the dry ingredients with the wet ingredients. Pour into the pan and bake for 45 minutes.

To make the frosting, using a blender, mix together all ingredients. Once the loaf has cooled, top with frosting and enjoy!

◆ ◆ ◆

Now, you are armed with all of the tools that you will need to improve your fertility with nutrition. Planning out your meals, with the help of the recipes included here and in chapter 5, will be a breeze, and you also know the importance of reducing stress and improving your support networks. Next, we will review what you need to know about toxins in our food and food environment that can impact fertility.

CHAPTER 8

Beyond Food: What You Need to Know About Toxins

We tend to think of a "food" as something that we can eat, and usually that thing is good for us (contains calories, and hopefully some nutrients). Some foods are known to be "less healthy," like ice cream and chips, whereas others are thought to be considered healthy options, like bananas and spinach. But there is more to it than that. Many seemingly healthy foods contain additives or ingredients that can be detrimental to having a baby. The problem is that it isn't always obvious when a food contains these additives. In this section, I want to talk about some of the things that can impact fertility that can be found in everyday foods, often due to environmental contamination. I want to help you to see that some of these potentially fertility-disrupting features of foods are rampant (and well hidden) in our food supply, but by being aware of them, you can avoid them and make better choices. Knowledge is power! Here you'll also find advice on food prep and storage, as well as helpful tips and guidelines to follow when shopping and eating out to ensure that your food is clean, safe, and, of course, fertility-friendly.

GMOs

Genetically modified organisms (GMOs), or genetically engineered foods, are basically crops (or organisms) that have had their DNA permanently changed by using genes from other plants or animals. To put it simply, scientists find a gene they like in one plant, and insert it into another plant to give the new plant some advantage. GMO crops are meant to benefit society by creating tastier and more nutritious foods, preventing disease, decreasing pesticide use, and increasing the food supply, among many other reasons.

A whopping 92 percent of corn grown in the United States is genetically engineered. In addition, 94 percent of soybeans and cotton (and thus, cottonseed oil) are also the product of GMOs. Considering the widespread use of these crops in what seems like every processed food, it's estimated that 75 percent, if not more, of processed foods contain GMO crops.

GMO isn't just limited to plants, either. Thus far, scientists have "safely" used this genetic engineering technology in cattle, pigs, chickens, goats, sheep, dogs, cats, fish, and even in rats and mice (for research purposes). As of this writing, the only approved genetically engineered animal on the market available for consumption is a genetically engineered Atlantic salmon, AquAdvantage Salmon.

To date, the research is inconclusive in regards to the effect of GMOs on male and female fertility. Most associations remain hypotheses, as scientists have not been able to find a strong connection in human studies. However, that doesn't mean that a link between GMOs and reproductive health doesn't exist. One hypothesis put forth by scientists is that GMOs influence endocrine metabolism, thus impacting fertility. Of the data that do exist from preclinical studies, there does seem to be some evidence that GMOs can disrupt fertility. One observational study in cows found that one year after GMO corn was introduced into the feed, the number of pregnancies decreased, and pathology reports found evidence of possible kidney damage. Other studies in rats have seen differences in body and organ weight or organ functioning, which certainly warrants further research.

If you don't want to risk it, there are definitely ways you can avoid GMO foods. Buy organic foods, and look for the USDA Organic label on packaged foods, since organic foods are not allowed to contain GMO ingredients. Some products may even be labeled "GMO free" and have a label from the Non-GMO Project and GMO Guard. Choose whole foods over processed, since GMOs are widely present in processed foods. Lastly, buy produce from the farmers' market when possible, and ask if they use GMO seeds on their farms or not.

Heavy Metals

There are many heavy metals that exist in the environment, but lead (Pb), cadmium (Cd), mercury (Hg), chromium (Cr), and arsenic (As) are particularly harmful to human health. These metals are especially toxic, because they can cause problems at very low concentrations. In addition, when they enter the body, they are stored in organs and bones instead of eliminated through urine.

Heavy metals tend to make their way into our bodies, like other contaminants, through food, water, air, or absorption through skin. Although heavy metals naturally occur in the environment, a major source of pollution is industrial use. Unfortunately, once these metals make it into the environment, they persist indefinitely.

You may be familiar with the recommendation to avoid fish containing high levels of mercury when pregnant or when trying to get pregnant. This is a good example of how heavy metals persist in the environment and can have an impact on human health. As mentioned, heavy metals accumulate in the body (even fish bodies), thus big predator fish such as swordfish and ahi have high levels of mercury due to eating lots of other fish that container smaller amounts of mercury. In regards to the health effects, mercury is a neurotoxin that can impact the memory, cognitive thinking, attention, language, and fine motor and visuospatial skills of a developing fetus.

Mercury impacts fertility through its disruption of the hypothalamus, pituitary, adrenal, and gonadal glands that release fertility-related hormones. As a result, we see disruptions in sperm production and erectile dysfunction in males, and menstrual disorders, premature menopause, and ovarian dysfunction in females.

Lead is toxic to almost all of our organs, and there are several ways in which lead impacts the reproductive system of both men and women. In women, menstrual disruptions, altered hormone production, spontaneous abortion, and delayed conception time are just a few ways in which lead toxicity affects female fertility and the ability to have a successful pregnancy. In men, there is evidence that lead can affect libido, sperm count and motility, and testosterone levels and even damage sperm DNA.

A wide variety of studies have found outcomes similar to those caused by lead and mercury for cadmium, chromium, and arsenic. Basically, changes in sex hormones, decreased sperm quality (such as sperm motility), menstrual irregularities, and adverse pregnancy outcomes arise from excess exposure to any of these heavy metals.

Because heavy metals are such potent endocrine disruptors, avoiding exposure is key if you want to get pregnant and have a successful pregnancy. The most common sources of exposure for these heavy metals are contaminated drinking water, industrial work sites, and lead paint, and, for mercury, predator fish such as king mackerel, swordfish, shark, orange roughy, tilefish, ahi, and bigeye tuna. The best thing you can do is test your drinking water, avoid fixing up a house that may have old lead paint, and avoid eating too much high-mercury fish. Since heavy metal tests aren't routine, your doctor may not test you unless there is reason to believe you have been exposed to high amounts.

Perchlorate

Perchlorate is an industrial chemical used mostly in rocket fuel, but it can also be found in fireworks, explosives, matches, flares, vehicle airbags, chlorine cleaners, pool chlorination chemicals, and some chewing tobacco. Perchlorate gets into our bodies mainly by eating or drinking food/beverages that have been contaminated with perchlorate or by chewing tobacco that contains perchlorate.

As you can probably imagine, this chemical definitely was not made to be in the food supply. Unfortunately, many of us are at risk of exposure and its toxic side effects. In the National Health and Nutrition Examination Survey in 2003–2004, CDC scientists found perchlorate in the urine of all 2,504 participants tested. So despite its intended purpose, perchlorate is clearly everywhere.

Perchlorate is known to affect the thyroid gland by disrupting uptake of iodine, and if one is exposed to high levels over time, it can cause hypothyroidism. According to the CDC, perchlorate can actually be used in a medical setting to treat a hyperactive thyroid.

However, when hypothyroidism results, it causes a variety of problems, including reduced fertility in males and females.

In women, hypothyroidism can lead to alteration of estrogen metabolism, menstrual irregularities, and disruptions in oocyte maturation and ovulation. In males, hypothyroidism can disrupt testosterone levels, reduce semen volume and sperm motility, and potentially lead to erectile dysfunction.

In order to fully understand and confirm the effects of perchlorate toxicity in humans, researchers extensively undertake animal studies. In several different species, researchers have found that perchlorate exposure negatively affects reproduction and fertility, in both long-term and short-term exposure. One study in rats found that in addition to altering thyroid functioning, perchlorate exposure also damaged testicular tissue.

If you're trying to get pregnant, being wary of your perchlorate exposure is essential. Not only is there plenty of research that shows it affects fertility, but once you're pregnant, disruptions in the thyroid could cause problems with your baby's neural development.

Although it can be difficult to avoid contaminated products (especially because typically we don't know they are contaminated), you should test your drinking water periodically for perchlorates. Use bottled water if you think your tap water may be contaminated. If you use well water, and you find that your well water has high levels of perchlorate, it is recommended to contact your local or state health agency or the CDC. In addition, it may be a good idea to get in touch with your doctor to discuss further steps. Discontinue use of chewing tobacco, and avoid igniting flares, fireworks, and matches in small, enclosed environments (i.e., inside your house or garage).

BPA

Bisphenol A (BPA) can be found in a variety of places and products. BPA is a chemical primarily produced for use in polycarbonate plastics and epoxy resins. Polycarbonate plastics are what you might find in food and drink packaging, as well as things we may eat or drink out of, such as reusable bottles (including infant bottles). Epoxy resins are typically manufactured for use in building or construction applications, but they can also be used in lacquers to coat metal products like food cans and water pipes. Other common sources of BPA include children's toys and the receipts you get from the grocery store.

Despite the wide use of BPA, most of what we're exposed to that ends up in the body comes from our diet. BPA often leaches from food and beverage storage containers, water bottles, plastic packaging, metal cans for canned foods, and even cardboard boxes that may have a protective lining. Temperature can affect BPA leaching, so leaving a water bottle in the sun or microwaving containers made from polycarbonate plastic would increase your chances of BPA exposure.

Studies show us that BPA is a strong endocrine disruptor, meaning it interferes with endocrine processes in the body. For example, BPA interacts with estrogen receptors and may have estrogen-like activity. This disruption has been shown to play a role in the pathogenesis of not only infertility in both males and females but also endocrine disorders such as polycystic ovarian syndrome (PCOS) and endometriosis.

In males exposed to BPA, we see a lower sperm cell production in addition to reduced motility and viability. In females, we see the development of endocrine disorders that reduce fertility (like PCOS) and poor oocyte development, meaning that BPA exposure could affect IVF outcomes as well.

Despite these findings, BPA exposure is widespread in the United States—CDC scientists tested the urine of 2,517 participants who took part in the National Health and Nutrition Examination Survey (NHANES) during 2003–2004 and found BPA in nearly every sample. This is partly due to the fact that the levels of BPA used in food packaging and other food applications are considered safe by the FDA. This brings up a question: If the FDA considers current BPA usage safe, do we really need to avoid it?

Although we can't disregard that not all studies show that BPA has an impact on human health, there is an overwhelming amount of evidence from animal studies and some human studies that say otherwise. To err on the side of safety, use containers or reusable bottles that say "BPA free," and increase your consumption of whole foods to avoid the use of packaged and canned foods. Avoid heating up polycarbonate plastics or leaving bottles in the sun, and store food in glass containers if possible.

Polychlorinated Biphenyls (PCBs)

Just like BPA, PCBs are another type of endocrine disrupter that confuses your body. Unlike BPA, PCBs are no longer produced; in fact, they haven't been made since 1977. Even though they aren't produced anymore, it's thought that more than half of PCBs previously created were released (from things like spills, improper disposal, and leaks) into the environment. Since these chemicals bind tightly to other types of residues, they are able to travel very long distances and have been found in the air, water, and soil all over the world, and unfortunately in our food chain.

Whether PCBs enter your body from food or contaminated drinking water, or even in the air you breathe, they are not eliminated well and can accumulate in your body, especially in your fatty tissues. Exposure to PCBs often happens when eating fish or meat that is contaminated. For example, smaller fish may ingest PCBs by eating plankton that have eaten PCBs, which then accumulate in the tissues. Then the larger fish eat the smaller fish and their absorbed PCBs, which is just one way these chemicals make it into our food supply. Carp and catfish are two that should be avoided since they have been found to have high levels.

Like many other chemicals, PCBs are associated with many reproductive issues. One study found that time to pregnancy was higher in women with the greatest amount of PCBs and, in couples undergoing IVF, those with higher levels of PCBs are less likely to become pregnant. Certain PCBs also negatively impact male fertility; exposure has been shown to alter sperm motility, volume and structure. There are associations between PCBs and the risk of endometriosis, which is a gynecologic disease. Although it is still very possible to become pregnant with this disease, it is more difficult. High blood levels of this chemical are associated with a significantly decreased ability to become pregnant as well as an increased rate of miscarriage.

So how can you try and avoid PCB exposure? Besides avoiding certain fish, stay away from older electrical equipment, cable insulation, oil-based paints, floor finishes and thermal insulation in order to help reduce the amount of contact you have with PCBs. Plasticizers added to paint and some rubber products also have been made with PCBs in the past. Check out the EPA website ,www.epa.gov/pcbs, to get a more detailed list as well as their trade names.

Phthalates

Phthalates are chemicals used ubiquitously to make plastics soft and flexible. They're used in a wide variety of products, from hairspray and detergent to pharmaceuticals. Phthalates are also in the food you eat, from fresh fruits and vegetables to fast food. That's not because they are naturally found in food though; phthalates get into the food supply because of food packaging and food-handling equipment, similarly to BPA. Phthalates can get into our bodies through ingestion, inhalation, or skin contact (such as playing with a plastic toy).

According to the FDA, it's not clear what effects phthalates have on human health. Like BPA, human exposure to phthalates is ubiquitous. Most likely due to the presence of phthalates in cosmetics, young women tend to have higher concentrations in their urine than do men. In addition, those who use medications with slow-release capsules may also be exposed to more phthalates than others. The Environmental Defense Fund (EDF) and public health agencies have submitted petitions to the FDA in the past two years to have a certain class of phthalates removed from food packaging, due to the evidence that they may no longer be considered safe.

Phthalates can act as endocrine disruptors, or in other words, hormone-mimicking chemicals. In laboratory animals, phthalates cause a variety of problems from birth defects to reproductive problems. More recently, researchers have come to find that certain classes of phthalates may also affect human reproduction or development. We know of one phthalate in particular (DEHP) that may even cause cancer.

In humans, we are seeing trends in phthalate exposure leading to reductions in fertility, including interfering with IVF success. For example, in 2018 researchers found that women undergoing IVF who had higher levels of phthalates in their urine also had lower levels of total, mature, and fertilized oocytes. Similarly, higher concentrations of phthalates were also found in the urine of women diagnosed with primary ovarian insufficiency. Researchers are finding that in general, infertile women have higher concentrations of phthalates in their bodies than fertile women.

Not so surprisingly, we see similar results in men. Basically, studies are finding that the more exposure a male has to phthalates (typically measured by the amount in urine), the more likely it is that the male will experience a decline in semen quality, including a decrease in sperm motility. One study also found that men with a BMI ≥ 25 may be even more susceptible to the possible health effects of phthalates.

Although phthalates are just about everywhere, there are ways in which you can avoid them to reduce your overall exposure. Just as you would to avoid BPA exposure, don't microwave food in plastic and be sure to opt for microwave-safe containers if you do. Avoid chewing on soft plastics or vinyls (like straws), and use only plastic/vinyl toothbrushes that are labeled "phthalate-free." Typically you can look inside the universal recycle label for this—if it contains the number 3 inside, as well as V or PVC underneath, the product contains phthalates. Lastly, research and support companies that make phthalate-free products such as cosmetics. Reading a label usually isn't enough. It is unlikely that you'll see "contains phthalates" on ingredient labels, so it's important to go the extra step and do your own research.

PFAS (perfluoroalkyl and polyfluoroalkyl substances)

PFAS is a very large group of chemicals used to make everyday products, similarly to phthalates. The utility of PFAS is vast—for example, you can find them in nonstick cookware, stain-resistant clothes and carpets, and in the foam of fire extinguishers.

Like BPA and phthalates, PFAS are widespread in the United States. Based on a CDC report, 97 percent of Americans have PFAS in their blood. In the early 2000s, certain PFAS were removed from consumer products, but the variety and number of new PFAS appears to be increasing (currently, more than 4,700 PFAS exist). In addition, it's unclear how long it takes PFAS to break down in the environment and it's possible that they may take years to leave the body.

In an effort to find out more about the health effects of these widespread chemicals, researchers have uncovered that in addition to affecting your ability to get pregnant, PFAS may also reduce birth weight and fetal growth, negatively affect cognition in children with prenatal exposure, and reduce the amount of time a woman is able to breastfeed her child.

According to the Natural Resources Defense Council, we are currently in a PFAS crisis because the drinking water of 6 million Americans is contaminated with unsafe levels of PFAS. Basically, PFAS are extremely hard to avoid. However, there are some things you can do to decrease your PFAS exposure.

According to the Environmental Working Group, you should cut back on fast food and microwave popcorn, use stainless steel or cast-iron cookware, avoid clothing or personal products that contain Gore-Tex or Teflon or "PTFE" or "FLUORO" ingredients, and skip the stain-repellent treatments for carpets, furniture, or shoes, because these often contain PFAS. Basically, fast-food containers, microwave popcorn bags, stain-resistant or water-repellant clothing, nonstick cookware, and many other products for personal and commercial use fall into these categories and should be avoided.

Pesticides and Herbicides

Although there is almost no way to completely steer clear of pesticides, avoiding them should be high on your priority list if you're trying to get pregnant. Studies have found that as blood levels of certain pesticides increase, fertility problems increase as well. Many pesticides have been banned in the United States (like DDT), but a lot of these older pesticides stay in the soil for years and years, and some are still used in other countries. Although there is a need for more research in humans, glyphosate, an herbicide used worldwide and found in products like Roundup may actually harm your reproductive health as well. The human data is still debated by many, but it is associated with lower sperm counts in male rodents, and shown to negatively impact uterine health as well. Although higher exposure has been shown to shorten gestation time in pregnant women, it is currently not viewed as toxic or an endocrine disruptor by the EPA. But, some argue that the impact of long-term, chronic exposure to this herbicide has on human health should continue to be tested, and it has been banned in several European countries. The laws regarding pesticide use are different across countries so it's hard to compare all these studies to each other. However, pesticides are rapidly metabolized in our body, and high levels of exposure prior to pregnancy have been negatively linked to fertility. Additionally, in women undergoing assisted reproduction, those who consumed high amounts of fruits and vegetables with pesticides had a lower chance of becoming pregnant and having a live birth, compared to those with lower intakes. But on a positive note, a recent study also found that following a diet with less pesticides increased the likelihood of becoming pregnant. Since eating more fruits and vegetables with lower pesticide residues is associated with better reproductive parameters, avoiding fruits and veggies is not recommended. But not to worry, they don't *all* have to be organic. While there is a decently long list of conventional produce that should be avoided, there is also a list of foods that do not have to be organic because they are relatively "clean." Asparagus, avocado cauliflower, carrots, grapefruit, mango, and pineapple are all examples of produce that has a lower pesticide residue, so you can opt for the non-organic variety of these if you like.

If fresh organic produce from the list of "dirty" foods is just too much of a financial strain, opt for the organic frozen varieties. They're just as nutritious and relatively cheaper! Plus the frozen spinach and kale is already cleaned—which saves *a lot* of prep time.

Unfortunately, pesticides aren't just found in fruits and vegetables. They are also detected in wheat, rice, cotton, flowers, and olives and olive oil, as well as in canola oil. Additionally, crops that are used as animal feed are also sprayed with pesticides, but at least the residues are not typically found in either meat or dairy products.

Smoking and Secondhand Smoke

Smoking is a bad habit with terrible consequences for your reproductive health. Cigarettes contain over 4,000 different chemicals, including heavy metals and polycyclic aromatic hydrocarbons (those same chemicals found in barbecued foods), all which are not helping your chances of getting pregnant. Smoking is a very hard habit to break, but it is worth it, especially if you want to become pregnant. Smoking increases your risk of spontaneous abortion and increases the time it takes to become pregnant. Not only do these chemicals damage the ovaries, contribute to oxidative stress and inflammation, and reduce sperm quality as well as function, but women who smoke may also enter menopause earlier than women who never have. Since it negatively impacts men and women, if you and/or your partner currently smoke, it's time to really try to quit. If you don't currently smoke—Great! Just make sure to stay away from secondhand smoke. Passive smoke can also negatively impact pregnancy and has been associated with higher rates of infertility and early menopause as well as lower rates of conception in women with PCOS. And keep this practice going especially if you do become pregnant. Prenatal secondhand smoke exposure has also been associated with delayed neurodevelopment as well as asthma and sudden infant death syndrome.

• •

A Word on Vaping

When vaping first came out, it was advertised as a safer alternative to smoking, and many young girls and pregnant women started smoking these devices instead of cigarettes. They smell a lot better, and they come in flavors like cupcake and chocolate, and although they expose a smoker to fewer toxic chemicals than traditional cigarettes, we are now learning that they aren't necessarily "safe." E-cigarettes and vape pens still deliver many chemicals, including nicotine, which is highly addictive. Although the research on the influence on fertility of vaping before conception is still in its early stages, the researching into the detrimental effects that nicotine has on reproduction is not, so it's probably a good idea to avoid e-cigarettes and vape pens. However, one study conducted in mice found that exposure to e-cigarettes impaired embryo implantation. Although there are still many gaps in the literature regarding the effects of vaping on health, it has been shown to increase inflammation. Since higher inflammation is associated with lower fertility rates, this alone should show that vaping is not as safe as it was once advertised to be. Plus, prenatal e-cigarette use is associated with increased risk of "small for gestational age" at birth, so it's likely safe to assume that avoiding these devices is a good idea.

• •

Marijuana and CBD

At this point in time, there are more than ten states across the country that have fully legalized marijuana, making it a lot more common and a less taboo topic to talk about. But, the relationship between smoking pot and getting pregnant is very complex, as some studies show that there is no negative impact on time of conception, while other studies show that there is. However, studies have found cannabis use to be associated with lower sperm concentrations, which would ultimately impact reproductive outcomes. Further, studies have also found that males who acutely and chronically use marijuana have had lower testosterone levels, and men and women who smoke marijuana had lower fertility rates. Conversely, a large study conducted found that using any marijuana while trying to conceive has no relationship to the time to get pregnant. However, this may not be the case in couples actively undergoing infertility treatment. No blanket statement can be made about the relationship of marijuana to reproductive health, but because receptors that cannabis binds to are found throughout the male and female reproductive systems, there is definitely a relationship between the two that needs to be further explored.

You might be wondering about cannabidiol (CBD). CBD is part of the marijuana plant that is touted as having medicinal properties but does not get you "high." Many people swear by CBD for reducing anxiety and promoting sleep, although research studies are limited. Some even suggest that CBD can help with fertility, mostly as a result of reducing anxiety and promoting sleep. However, research studies have not backed this up, and of the studies that are out there, the research seems to suggest that chronic use of CBD can have a negative effect on the reproductive health of males.

Air Pollution

Depending on where you live, air pollution can be a major problem for your health. Not only is it positively associated with respiratory issues, cancer, and mental health problems, but it's also detrimental for fertility. Ozone, which comes from things like car exhaust, factory fumes and gasoline can be found inside and outside, and contributes to many reproductive problems, including higher risk of stillbirth. Traffic-related pollutants are also associated with increased risk of IVF failure in the early phases, as well as higher risk of miscarriage and infertility. Pollution has the ability to interfere with endocrine and reproductive processes and can increase the time it takes for people to become pregnant; it also contributes to increased levels of oxidative stress in the body, which harms ovarian function.

Even though face masks are common in some parts of the country, and world, not everyone wants to wear one. When tested, many of the face masks that claim to keep out pollution don't do a very good job, mainly since they don't fit people's faces very well. But, if you do decide to wear a mask, make sure it fits your face properly and has been tested to keep out particulate matter.

In addition to a proper mask, one study conducted in women who were using assisted reproductive technology found that supplementing with folate may have a protective effect on fertility outcomes against exposure to nitrogen dioxide, a common air pollutant.

Besides a well-fitting face mask, and possibly folate (although additional research is needed), here are some things to keep in mind that can help you decrease the amount of pollution you breathe in:

1. Don't exercise outside during rush hour, and avoid working out by main roads.

2. Walk down a quieter street (assuming it's safe); fewer cars means less pollution.

3. Do not burn trash or plastic in a fireplace; you should burn wood only.

4. If you have an old stove, think about replacing it with one that is approved by the EPA.

5. Download an air-quality app and follow the advice that it gives!

6. When cleaning, don't mix products, use gloves, and make sure the area is well ventilated.

7. Make sure your carbon monoxide alarm is working

8. Eat a healthy diet with a variety of fruits and vegetables—the antioxidants help mitigate the negative effects of the pollution.

Parabens

Here's another endocrine disrupting chemical to add to the list. Parabens are a group of industrial chemicals that are added to many cosmetics as preservatives. They can also be found in other products like food and medicine, which make exposure quite likely. These chemicals are added to help prevent the growth of mold and bacteria, especially in products with high water content like shampoos and moisturizers, but they are absorbed through the skin, and once in the body can interfere with many different hormones.

Even though there are many different parabens to be on the lookout for, some of the most common parabens added to products are methylparaben, propylparaben, butylparaben, and ethylparaben. The good news is that product labels must indicate if these chemicals are present in the product, so they are easier to spot.

Depending on where you live, certain parabens are no longer allowed to be added to products and many large companies are committed to excluding certain ones from being added to their own products. Parabens are mainly eliminated from the body, however they also accumulate in the fat tissue, so avoiding certain products will significantly reduce your future exposure.

It's a good idea to reduce your exposure to these chemicals, especially if you're actively trying to get pregnant. Animal studies have shown that parabens have the ability to decrease ovarian weight and structure, and also bind with estrogen receptors. Exposure has also been associated with a shorter menstrual cycle and parabens even affect hormone metabolism by interacting with different receptors. Parabens have been shown to affect glucose levels in women at high risk of gestational diabetes in the first trimester. In fact, during the first trimester, urinary ethylparaben was significantly associated with future diagnosis of gestational diabetes. However, it is important to note that other studies have found no negative correlation between becoming pregnant and paraben exposure, so additional work on this topic is needed. In the meantime, reducing your exposure can't hurt. Start reading the ingredient labels of your cosmetics and lotions, and look for companies that make products that are labeled as "Paraben Free." Besides lotions, be mindful of the food that you're eating also. Certain foods have parabens added to them for preservation purposes. Many foods that may have parabens are ones that you should try and avoid anyway, including beers, frozen dairy products, sodas, and processed foods.

Supplements

Taking supplements can be a healthy part of your diet. Not all of the nutrients that we need are readily available from the foods we are eating, in part, because we don't always eat the right foods. But nutrient deficiency isn't all due to lifestyle: Due to changes in our soil and farming practices, many of the vegetables and fruits we grow aren't as nutrient dense as they used to be. For example, many of the new breeds of fruits and vegetables that are grown do not have the same amount of key vitamins like B and C when compared to fifty years ago. Because crops are grown a lot faster nowadays, in addition to being bigger, they don't seem to absorb nutrients from the soil as well as they used to. So, in some cases, many fruits and veggies aren't providing the amount of essential vitamins and minerals as you assume they are, and this, coupled with a poor overall diet quality, has led to more deficiencies. Vitamin deficiencies negatively impact many disease states ranging from dermatological illnesses to bone diseases and diabetes. Deficiencies of certain vitamins also play a role in fertility; for example, women with infertility had higher rates of suboptimal vitamin D compared to the average population, and women undergoing IVF with higher levels of vitamin D were more likely to have a clinical pregnancy.

Often supplementation is warranted (like to ensure that you're getting enough iron and folate before and throughout pregnancy), however many times people just take a vitamin because they read somewhere that they "should" when in reality they may not need it, and it may actually be doing more harm than good. Since there is not much government oversight when it comes to the multibillion-dollar supplement industry, there is a lot of room for things to go wrong. Heavy metals, toxic chemicals, and even bacteria have been found in supplements. In fact, one recent study that tested over twenty-five different prenatal vitamins found toxic levels of lead, arsenic, and titanium in them. This is not to say that all vitamins are dangerous, there are many high quality ones that are available—it's just important to do some research before starting to supplement. A good place to make sure that your vitamins are not contaminated, and actually have the amount of nutrients that is touted on the label (often those numbers are not actually true representations) is to review it at Consumer Labs website. Additionally, when a pharmacy or facility has been found to have contamination, the FDA will issue a press release on their website, which is another good resource just to make sure that what you are supplementing with isn't hurting you more than helping you.

◆ ◆ ◆

Having a baby is one of the greatest journeys you will embark on. No matter where you are in the journey, having a healthy diet will help, and I hope that the information in this book has helped you to see that you can control more than you think.

References

Chapter 1: So You Want to Have a Baby . . .

Agency for Toxic Substances and Disease Registry. (1999) Public Health Statement for Mercury. Retrieved from www.atsdr.cdc.gov/phs/phs.asp?id=112&tid=24 October 31, 2019.

Akmal M., Qadri J.Q., Al-Waili N.S., Thangal S., Hag A., Saloom K.Y. (2006) Improvement in semen quality after oral supplementation of vitamin C. *Journal of Medicinal Food*, 9(3): 440–442.

Center for Science in the Public Interest. (2016) Seeing Red. Retrieved from cspinet.org/sites/default/files/attachment/Seeing percent20Red.pdf October 31, 2019.

Centers for Disease Control and Prevention. (2019) Infertility FAQs. Retrieved from www.cdc.gov/reproductivehealth/infertility/index.htm October 30, 2019.

Centers for Disease Control and Prevention. (2019) Vital Statistics Rapid Release. Retrieved from www.cdc.gov/nchs/data/vsrr/vsrr-007-508.pdf October 30, 2019.

Chai W., Morimoto Y., Cooney R.V., et al. (2017) Dietary red and processed meat intake and markers of adiposity and inflammation: The multiethnic cohort study. *Journal of the American College of Nutrition*, 36(5): 378–385.

Chavarro J.E., Rich-Edwards J.W., Rosner B.A., Willet W.C. (2007) Diet and lifestyle in the prevention of ovulatory disorder infertility. *Obstetrics and Gynecology*, 110(5): 1050–1058.

Child Trends. (2019) Fertility and Birth Rates. Retrieved from www.childtrends.org/indicators/fertility-and-birth-rates October 30, 2019.

Chiu Y.H., Karmon A.E., Gaskins A.J., et al. (2018) Serum omega-3 fatty acids and treatment outcomes among women undergoing assisted reproduction. *Human Reproduction*, 33(1): 156–165.

Dag Z.O., Dilbaz B. (2015) Impact of obesity on infertility in women. *Journal of the Turkish-German Gynecological Association*, 16(2): 111–117.

Eunice Kennedy Shriver National Institute of Child Health and Human Development. (2017) What Causes Amenorrhea? Retrieved from www.nichd.nih.gov/health/topics/amenorrhea/conditioninfo/causes October 30, 2019.

Fallah A., Mohammad-Hasani A., Colagar A.H. (2018) Zinc is an essential element for male fertility: A review of Zn roles in men's health, germination, sperm quality, and fertilization. *Journal of Reproduction and Infertility*, 19(2): 69–81.

Gaskins A.J., Afeiche M., Wright D.L., et al. (2015) Dietary folate and reproductive success among women undergoing assisted reproduction. *Obstetrics and Gynecology*, 124(4): 801–809.

Halpern G., Braga D.P., Setti A.S., Figueira R.C., Iaconeli Jr. A., Borges Jr. E. (2016) Artificial sweeteners: Do they bear an infertility risk? *Fertility and Sterility*, 106(3): e263.

Hambidge K.M., Krebs N.F. (2018) Strategies for optimizing maternal nutrition to promote infant development. *Reproductive Health*, 15: 87.

Iamsaard S., Sukhorum W., Samrid R., et al. (2014) The sensitivity of male rat reproductive organs to monosodium glutamate. *Acta Medica Academica*, 43(1): 3–9.

Moslemi M.K., Tavanbakhsh S. (2011) Selenium-vitamin E supplementation in infertile men: Effects on semen parameters and pregnancy rate. *International Journal of General Medicine*, 4: 99–104.

National Center for Complementary and Integrative Health. (2016) Flaxseed and flaxseed oil. Retrieved from nccih.nih.gov/health/flaxseed/ataglance.htm October 26, 2019.

Nerin C., Canellas E., Vera P., et al. (2018) A common surfactant used in food packaging found to be toxic for reproduction in mammals. *Food and Chemical Toxicology*, 113: 115–124.

Office on Women's Health. (2019) Infertility. Retrieved from www.womenshealth.gov/a-z-topics/infertility October 30, 2019.

Sindelar J.J., Milkowski A.L. (2012) Human safety controversies surrounding nitrate and nitrite in the diet. *Nitric Oxide*, 26(4): 259–266.

Stephenson J., Heslehurst N., Hall J., et al (2018) Before the beginning: Nutrition and lifestyle in the preconception period and its importance for future health. *Lancet*, 391(10132): 1830–1841.

Vannuccini S., Clifton V.L., Fraser I.S., et al. (2016) Infertility and reproductive disorders: Impact of hormonal and inflammatory mechanisms on pregnancy outcome. *Human Reproduction Update*, 22(1): 104–115.

Weiss G., Goldsmith L.T., Taylor R.N., Bellet D., Taylor H.S. (2011) Inflammation in reproductive disorders. *Reproductive Sciences*, 16(2): 216–229.

Chapter 2: The Importance of Diet for a Healthy Pregnancy

Belan M., Harnois-Leblanc S., Laferrere B., Baillargeon J. (2018). Optimizing reproductive health in women with obesity and infertility. *Canadian Medical Association Journal*, 190(24): E742–E745.

Bueno N.B., de Melo I.S., de Oliveria S.L., da Rocha Ataide T. (2013) Very-low-carbohydrate ketogenic diet v. low-fat diet for long-term weight loss: A meta-analysis of randomised controlled trials. *British Journal of Nutrition*, 110(7): 1178–1187.

Bygren L.O., Kaati G., Edvinsson S. (2001) Longevity determined by paternal ancestors' nutrition during their slow growth period. *Acta Biotheoretica*, 49: 53–59.

Cabler S,, Agarwal A., Flint M., Du Plessis S.S. (2010) Obesity: Modern man's fertility nemesis. *Asian Journal of Andrology*, 12(4): 480–489.

Centers for Disease Control and Prevention. (2016) Birth Expectations of U.S. Women Aged 15–44. Retrieved from www.cdc.gov/nchs/products/databriefs/db260.htm October 31, 2019.

Centers for Disease Control and Prevention. Healthy Weight: The Health Effects of Overweight and Obesity. Retrieved from www.cdc.gov/healthyweight/effects/index.html, November 2, 2019.

Centers for Disease Control and Prevention. (2016) Infertility. Retrieved from www.cdc.gov/nchs/fastats/infertility.htm October 30, 2019.

Centers for Disease Control and Prevention. National Center for Health Statistics Overweight and Obese. Retrieved from www.cdc.gov/nchs/fastats/obesity-overweight.htm November 2, 2019.

Colhan I., Erdem E., Usta A., Karacan M. (2018) The effects of obesity and bariatric surgery on fertility. *Journal of Obstetrics & Gynecology*, 28(2): 65–74.

de Rooij S.R., Painter R.C., Holleman F., Bossuyt P.M., Roseboom T.J. (2007) The metabolic syndrome in adults prenatally exposed to the Dutch famine. *American Journal of Clinical Nutrition*, 86: 1219–1224.

de Rooij S.R., Painter R.C., Roseboom T.J. (2006) Glucose tolerance at age 58 and the decline of glucose tolerance in comparison with age 50 in people prenatally exposed to the Dutch famine. *Diabetologia*, 49: 637–643.

Dunson D.B., Colombo B., Baird D.D. (2002) Changes with age in the level and duration of fertility in the menstrual cycle. *Human Reproduction*, 17(5): 1399–1403.

Efrat M., Stein A., Pinkas H., Unger R., Birk R. (2018) Dietary patterns are positively associated with semen quality. *Andrology*, 109(5): 809–816.

Eunice Kennedy Shriver National Institute of Child Health and Human Development. (2017) What Lifestyle and Environmental Factors May Be Involved With Infertility in Females and Males? Retrieved from www.nichd.nih.gov/health/topics/infertility/conditioninfo/causes/lifestyle November 2, 2019.

Fallah A., Mohammad-Hasani A., Colaga A.H. (2018). Zinc is an essential element for male fertility: A review of Zn roles in men's health, germination, sperm quality and fertilization. *Journal of Reproduction & Infertility*, 19(2): 69–81.

Fleming T.P., Eckert J.J., Denisenko O. (2017) The role of maternal nutrition during the periconceptional period and its effect on offspring phenotype. *Advances in Experimental Medicine and Biology*, 1014: 87–105.

Gaskins A.J., Chavarro J.E. (2018) Diet and fertility: A review. *American Journal of Obstetrics and Gynecology*, 218(4): 379–389.

Glockner G., Seralini G. (2016). Pathology reports on the first cows fed with Bt175 maize (1997–2002). *Scholarly Journal of Agricultural Science*, 6(1): 1–8.

Guerrero-Bosagna C., Skinner M.K. (2014) Environmental epigenetics and effects on male fertility. *Advances in Experimental Medicine and Biology*, 791: 67–81.

Guo D., Xu M., Zhou Q., Wu C., Ju R., Dai J. (2019) Is low body mass index a risk factor for semen quality? A PRISMA-compliant meta-analysis. *Medicine (Baltimore)*, 98(32): e16677.

Hamilton B.E., Martin J.A., Sutton P.D. (2004) Births: Preliminary data for 2003. *National Vital Statistics Reports*, 53(9): 1–7.

Hohos N.M., Cho K.J., Swindle D.C., Skaznik-Wikiel M.E. (2018). High-fat diet exposure, regardless of induction of obesity, is associated with altered expression of genes critical to normal ovulatory function. *Molecular and Cellular Endocrinology*, 470: 199–207.

Imam M.U., Ismail M. (2017) The impact of traditional food and lifestyle behavior on epigenetic burden of chronic disease. *Global Challenges*,1(8): 1700043.

Kumar S. (2018). Occupational and environmental exposure to lead and reproductive health impairment: Overview. *Indian Journal of Occupational & Environmental Medicine*, 22(3): 128–137.

Ly L., Chan D., Aarabi M., et al. (2017) Intergenerational impact of paternal lifetime exposures to both folic acid deficiency and supplementation on reproductive outcomes and imprinted gene methylation. *Molecular Human Reproduction*, 23(7): 461–477.

Morris M.C., Tangney C.C., Wang Y., Sacks F.M., Bennett D.A., Aggarwal N.T. (2015) MIND diet associated with reduced incidence of Alzheimer's disease. *Alzheimer's Dementia*, 11(9): 1107–1014.

Painter R.C., de Rooij S.R., Bossuyt P.M., et al. (2006) A possible link between prenatal exposure to famine and breast cancer: A preliminary study. *American Journal of Human Biology*, 18: 853–856.

Painter R.C., de Rooij S.R., Bossuyt P.M., et al. (2006) Early onset of coronary artery disease after prenatal exposure to the Dutch famine. *American Journal of Clinical Nutrition*, 84: 322–327.

Painter R.C., Osmond C., Gluckman P., et al. (2008) Transgenerational effects of prenatal exposure to the Dutch famine on neonatal adiposity and health in later life. *BJOG; An International Journal of Obstetrics & Gynecology*, 115: 1243–1249.

Pandey S., Pandey S., Maheshwari A., Bhattacharya S. (2010). The impact of female obesity on the outcome of fertility treatment. *Journal of Human Reproductive Sciences*. 3(2): 62–67.

Panth N., Gavarkovs A., Tamez M., Mattei J. (2018) The influence of diet on fertility and the implications for public health nutrition in the United States. *Frontiers in Public Health*, 6: 211.

Pembrey M.E., Bygren L.O., Kaati G., et al. (2006) Sex-specific, male-line transgenerational responses in humans. *European Journal of Human Genetics*, 14: 159–166.

Roseboom T., de Rooij S., Painter R. (2006) The Dutch famine and its long-term consequences for adult health. *Early Human Development*, 82: 485–491.

Roseboom T.J., Painter R.C., van Abeelen A.F., Veenendaal M.V., de Rooij S.R. (2011). Hungry in the womb: What are the consequences? Lessons from the Dutch famine. *Maturitas*, 70: 141–145.

Salas-Huetos A., Bullo M., Salas-Salvado J. (2017). Dietary patterns, foods and nutrients in male fertility parameters and fecundability: A systematic review of observational studies. *Human Reproduction Update*, 23(4): 371–389.

Salas-Huetos A., Rosique-Esteban N., Becerra-Tomas N., et al. (2018). Effect of nutrients and dietary supplements on sperm quality parameters: A systematic review and meta-analysis of randomized clinical trials. *Advances in Nutrition*, 9(6): 833–848.

Schagdarsurengin U., Steger K. (2016) Epigenetics in male reproduction: Effect of paternal diet on sperm quality and offspring health. *Nature Reviews Urology*, 13(10): 584–595.

Sedgh G., Singh S., Hussain R. (2014) Intended and unintended pregnancies worldwide in 2010 and recent trends. *Studies in Family Planning*, 45(3): 301–314.

Shreenath, A.P., Dooley J. (2019). Selenium Deficiency. [Updated 2019 Jun 3]. In: StatPearls [Internet]. Treasure Island (FL): StatPearls Publishing. Retrieved from www.ncbi.nlm.nih.gov/books/NBK482260/ November 2, 2019.

Silvestris E., Lovero D., Palmirotta R. (2019). Nutrition and female fertility: An independent correlation. *Frontiers in Endocrinology*, 10: 346.

Simone N., Gratta M., Scambia G. (2018). Is there a linkage between celiac disease and adverse pregnancy outcomes? *Clinical Gastroenterologist International*, 1(1004): 7–9.

Statovci D., Aquilera M., MacSharry J., Melgar S. (2017) The impact of Western diet and nutrients on the microbiota and immune response at mucosal interfaces. *Frontiers in Immunology*, 8: 838.

Tabler J., Utz R.L., Smith K.R., Hanson H.A., Geist C. (2018). Variation in reproductive outcomes of women with histories of bulimia nervosa, anorexia nervosa, or eating disorder not otherwise specified relative to the general population closest-aged sisters. *International Journal of Eating Disorders*, 51(2): 102–111.

United States Department of Health and Human Services. Office on Women's Health. Weight, Fertility and Pregnancy. Retrieved from www.womenshealth.gov/healthy-weight/weight-fertility-and-pregnancy November 2 , 2019.

Zain M.M., Norman R.J. (2008). Impact of obesity on female fertility and fertility treatment. *Women's Health*, 4(2): 183–194.

Zhou Y., Shi Y., Wan Y., Ye Z.W., Liu Q. (2017) Why the Mediterranean diet lowers the risk of heart disease. *European Journal of Preventative Cardiology*, 24(16): 1788–1789.

Chapter 3: Key Nutrients for Fertility

Abbaspour N., Hurrell R., Kelishadi R. (2014) Review on iron and its importance for human health. *Journal of Research in Medical Sciences*, 19(2): 164–174.

Abraham G.E. (1983) Nutritional factors in the etiology of the premenstrual tension syndromes. *The Journal of Reproductive Medicine*, 28(7): 446–464.

Aghajafari F., Nagulesapillai T., Ronksley P.E., Tough S.C., O'Beirne M., Rabi D.M. (2013) Association between maternal serum 25-hydroxyvitamin D level and pregnancy and neonatal outcomes: Systematic review and meta-analysis of observational studies. *British Medical Journal*, 346: f1169.

Akmal M., Qadri J.Q., Al-Aili N.S., Thangal S., Hag A., Saloom K.Y. (2006) Improvement in human semen quality after oral supplementation of vitamin C. *Journal of Medicinal Food*, 9(3): 440–442.

Al-Kunani A.S., Knight R., Haswell S.J., Thompson J.W., Lindow S.W. (2001) The selenium status of women with a history of recurrent miscarriage. *BJOG: An International Journal of Obstetrics and Gynecology*, 108(10): 1094–1097.

Anihani S.A. (2017) A systematic review evaluating the effect of vitamin B_6 on semen quality. *Urology Journal*, 30: 1–5.

Austin D.W., Spolding B., Gondalia S., et al. (2014) Genetic variation associated with hypersensitivity to mercury. *Toxicology International*, 21(3): 236–241.

Azizollahi G., Azizollahi S., Babaei H., et al. (2013) Effects of supplement therapy on sperm parameters, protamine content and acrosomal integrity of varicocelectomized subjects. *Journal of Assisted Reproduction and Genetics*, 30(4): 593–599.

Barrera D., Avila E., Hernández G. (2007) Estradiol and progesterone synthesis in human placenta is stimulated by calcitriol. *The Journal of Steroid Biochemistry and Molecular Biology*, 103(3–5): 529–532.

Barrie S.A., Wright J.V., Pizzomo J.E., Kutter E., Barron P.C. (1987) Comparative absorption of zinc picolinate, zinc citrate and zinc gluconate in humans. *Agents and Actions*, 21(1–2): 223–228.

Bennett M. (2001) Vitamin B_{12} deficiency, infertility and recurrent fetal loss. *Journal of Reproductive Medicine*, 46(3): 209–212.

Bergen N.E., Jaddoe V.W., Timmermans S., et al. (2012) Homocysteine and folate concentrations in early pregnancy and the risk of adverse pregnancy outcomes: The Generation R Study. *BJOG: An International Journal of Obstetrics and Gynaecology*, 119: 739–751.

Björn-Rasmussen E., Hallberg L., Isaksson B., Arvidsson B. (1974) Food iron absorption in man. Applications of the two-pool extrinsic tag method to measure heme and nonheme iron absorption from the whole diet. *The Journal of Clinical Investigation*, 53(1): 247–255.

Bliss R.M. (2004) Lack energy? Maybe it's your magnesium level. *Agricultural Research*, 52(5): 8.

Bloom M.S., Louis G.M., Sundaram R., Kostyniak P.J., Jain J. (2011) Associations between blood metals and fecundity among women residing in New York State. *Reproductive Toxicology*, 31(2): 158–163.

Boxmeer J.C., Smit M., Utomo E., et al. (2009) Low folate in seminal plasma is associated with increased sperm DNA damage. *Fertility and Sterility*, 92(2): 548–556.

Boyles A.L., Billups A.V., Deak K.L., et al. (2006). Neural tube defects and folate pathway genes: Family-based association tests of gene–gene and gene–environment interactions. *Environmental Health Perspectives*, 114: 1547–1552.

Brannon P.M., Picciano M.F. (2011) Vitamin D in pregnancy and lactation in humans. *Annual Review of Nutrition*, 31: 89–115.

Caffrey A., Irwin R.E., McNulty H., et al. (2018) Gene-specific DNA methylation in newborns in response to folic acid supplementation during the second and third trimesters of pregnancy: Epigenetic analysis from a randomized controlled trial. *American Journal of Clinical Nutrition*, 107: 566–575.

Calvo M.S., Whiting S.J., Barton C.N. (2004) Vitamin D fortification in the United States and Canada: Current status and data needs. *American Journal of Clinical Nutrition*, 80: 1710S-1716S.

Ceko M.J., Hummitzsch K., Hatzirodos N., et al. (2015) X-Ray fluorescence imaging and other analyses identify selenium and GPX1 as important in female reproductive function. *Metallomics*, 7(1): 71–82.

Centers for Disease Control and Prevention (2017) Folic acid fortification and supplementation. Retrieved from www.cdc.gov/ncbddd/folicacid/faqs/faqs-fortification.html November 6, 2019.

Cepeda-Lopez A.C., Melse A., Zimmermann M.B., Herter-Aeberli I. (2015) In overweight and obese women, dietary iron absorption is reduced and the enhancement of iron absorption by ascorbic acid is one-half that in normal-weight women. *American Journal of Clinical Nutrition,* 102: 1389–1397.

Chavarro J.E., Rich-Edwards J.W., Rosner B.A., Willett W.C. (2006) Iron intake and risk of ovulatory infertility. *Obstetrics & Gynecology,* 108(5): 1145–1152.

Chavarro J.E., Rich-Edwards J.W., Rosner B.A., Willett W.C. (2008) Use of multivitamins, intake of B vitamins, and risk of ovulatory infertility. *Fertility and Sterility,* 89(3): 668–676.

Chen J., Lan J., Liu D., et al. (2017) Ascorbic acid promotes the stemness of corneal epithelial stem/progenitor cells and accelerates epithelial wound healing in the cornea. *Stem Cells Translational Medicine,* 6(5): 1356–1365.

Cook J.D., Monsen E.R. (1977) Vitamin C, the common cold, and iron absorption. *The American Journal of Clinical Nutrition,* 30(2): 235–241.

Cook J.D., Reddy M.B. (2001) Effect of ascorbic acid intake on nonheme-iron absorption from a complete diet. *The American Journal of Clinical Nutrition,* 73(1): 93–98.

Czeizel A.E., Dudas, I. (1992) Prevention of the first occurrence of neural-tube defects by periconceptional vitamin supplementation. *New England Journal of Medicine,* 327: 1832–1835.

da Silva V.R., Hausman D.B., Kauwell G.P., et al. (2013) Obesity affects short-term folate pharmacokinetics in women of childbearing age. *International Journal of Obesity (London)*, 37(12): 1608–1610.

Dawson E.B., Harris W.A., Teter M.C., Powell L.C. (1992) Effect of ascorbic acid supplementation on the sperm quality of smokers. *Fertility and Sterility*, 58(5): 1034–1039.

De Vilbiss E.A., Gardner R.M., Newschaffer C.J., et al. (2015) Maternal folate status as a risk factor for autism spectrum disorders: A review of existing evidence. *British Journal of Nutrition*, 114: 663–672.

Di Nicolantonio J.J., McCarty M.F., O'Keefe J.H. (2017) Decreased magnesium status may mediate the increased cardiovascular risk associated with calcium supplementation. *Open Heart*, 4(1): e000617.

Doll H., Brown S., Thurston A., Vessey M. (1989) Pyridoxine (vitamin B_6) and the premenstrual syndrome: A randomized crossover trial. *The Journal of the Royal College of General Practitioners*, 39 (326): 364–368.

Dyckner T., Webster P.O. (1983) Effect of magnesium on blood pressure. *British Medical Journal*, 286(6381): 1847–1849.

Eby G.A., Eby K.L. (2006) Rapid recovery from major depression using magnesium treatment. *Medical Hypotheses*, 67(2): 362–370.

Eby G.A., Eby K.L. (2010) Magnesium for treatment-resistant depression: A review and hypothesis. *Medical Hypotheses*, 74(4): 649–660.

Eilander A., Hundscheid D.C., Osendarp S.J., Transler C., Zock P.L. (2007) Effects of n-3 long chain polyunsaturated fatty acid supplementation on visual and cognitive development throughout childhood: A review of human studies. *Prostaglandins, Leukotrines and Essential Fatty Acids*, 76: 189–203.

El-Khashab E.K., Hamdy A.M., Maher K.M., Fouad M.A., Abbas G.Z. (2013) Effect of maternal vitamin A deficiency during pregnancy on neonatal kidney size. *Journal of Perinatal Medicine*, 41(2): 199–203.

Esmaeili V., Shahverdi A.H., Moghadasian M.H., Alizadeh A.R. (2015) Dietary fatty acids affect semen quality: A review. *Andrology*, 3: 450–461.

Flohe L. (2007) Selenium in mammalian spermiogenesis. *Biological Chemistry*, 388: 987–995.

Frey S.K., Vogel S. (2011) Vitamin A metabolism and adipose tissue biology. *Nutrients*, 3(1): 27–39.

Garcia-Casal M.N., Layrisse M., Solano L., et al. (1998) Vitamin A and beta carotene can improve nonheme iron absorption from rice, wheat and corn by humans. *Journal of Nutrition*, 128(3): 646–650.

Gerster H. (1998) Can adults adequately convert alpha-linolenic acid (18:3n-3) to eicosapentaenoic acid (20:5n-3) and docosahexaenoic acid (22:6n-3)? *International Journal for Vitamin and Nutrition Research*, 68(3): 159–173.

Golden B.E., Golden M.H.N. (1981) Effect of zinc supplementation on the dietary intake, rate of weight gain, and energy cost of tissue deposition in children recovering from severe malnutrition. *The American Journal of Clinical Nutrition*, 34(5): 900–908.

Golden M.H.N. (1988) The Role of Individual Nutrient Deficiencies in Growth Retardation of Children as Exemplified by Zinc and Protein. Nestle Nutrition Workshop Series, vol.14. Nestec Ltd., Vevey/Raven Press Ltd., New York.

Gupta R.K. Ganfoliya S.S., Singh N.K. (2015) Reduction of phytic acid and enhancement of bioavailable micronutrients in food grains. *Journal of Food Science and Technology*, 52(2): 676–684.

Hallberg L., Hulthen L. (2000) Prediction of dietary iron absorption: An algorithm for calculating absorption and bioavailability of dietary iron. *American Journal of Clinical Nutrition*, 71(5): 1147–1160.

Hammoud A.O., Meikle A.W., Peterson C.M., Stanford J., Gibson M., Carrell D.T. (2012) Association of 25-hydroxy-vitamin D levels with semen and hormonal parameters. *Asian Journal of Andrology*, 14(6): 855–859.

Hammond B.R. (2013) Carotenoids. *Advances in Nutrition*, 4(4): 474–476.

Helland I.B., Smith L., Saarem K., Saugstad O.D., Drevon C.A. (2003) Maternal supplementation with very long chain n-3 fatty acids during pregnancy and lactation augments children's IQ at 4 years of age. *Pediatrics*, 111(1): e39–44.

Henkel R., Baldauf C., Bittner J., Weidner W., Miska W. (2001) Elimination of zinc from the flagella of spermatozoa during epididymal transit is important for motility. *Reproductive Technologies*, 10(5): 280–285.

Henmi H., Endo T., Kitajima Y., Manase K., Hata H., Kudo R. (2003) Effect of ascorbic acid supplementation on serum progesterone levels in patients with a luteal phase defect. *Fertility and Sterility*, 80(2): 459–461.

Horimoto Y., Lim L.T. (2017) Effects of different proteases on iron absorption property of egg white hydrolysates. *Food Research International*, 95: 108–116.

Howard J.M., Davies S., Hunnisett A. (1994) Red cell magnesium and glutathione perioxidase in infertile women—effects of oral supplementation with magnesium and selenium. *Magnesium Research*, 7(1): 49–57.

Hurrell R., Egli I. (2010) Iron bioavailability and dietary reference values. *The American Journal of Clinical Nutrition*, 91(5): 1461S-1467S.

Institute of Medicine. Food and Nutrition Board. (1998) Dietary Reference Intakes: Thiamin, Riboflavin, Niacin, Vitamin B_6, Folate, Vitamin B_{12}, Pantothenic Acid, Biotin, and Choline. Washington, DC: National Academy Press.

Irvine D.S. (1996) Glutathione as a treatment for male infertility. *Reviews of Reproduction*, 1, 6–12.

Iwasaki A., Hosaka M., Kinoshita Y., et al. (2003) Result of long-term methylcobalamin treatment for male infertility. *Japanese Journal of Fertility and Sterility*, 48: 119–124.

Jensen M.B., Bjerrum P.J., Jessen T.E. (2011) Vitamin D is positively associated with sperm motility and increases intracellular calcium in human spermatozoa. *Human Reproduction*, 26(6): 1307–1317.

Kaiser L., Allen L.H. (2008) Position of the American Dietetic Association: Nutrition and lifestyle for a healthy pregnancy outcome. *Journal of the American Dietetic Association*, 108: 553–61.

Kobayashi Y., Wakasugi E., Yasui R., Kuwahata M. (2015) Egg yolk protein delays recovery while ovalbumin is useful in recovery from iron deficiency anemia. *Nutrients*, 7(6): 4792–4803.

Leitzmann M.F., Stampfer M.J., Wu K., Colditz G.A., Willett W.C., Giovannucci E.L. (2003) Zinc supplement use and risk of prostate cancer. *Journal of the National Cancer Institute*, 95(13): 1004–1007.

Li W.X., Dai S.X., Zheng J.J., Liu J.Q., Huang J.F. (2015) Homocysteine metabolism gene polymorphisms (MTHFR C677T, MTHFR A1298C, MTR A2756G and MTRR A66G) jointly elevate the risk of folate deficiency. *Nutrients*, 7(8): 6670–6687.

Lombardi-Boccia G., Martinez-Dominguez B., Aguzzi A. (2002) Total heme and non-heme iron in raw and cooked meats. *Journal of Food Science*, 67: 1738–1741.

Lopez H.W., Leenhardt F., Coudray C., Remesy C. (2002) Minerals and phytic acid interactions: Is it a real problem for human nutrition? *International Journal of Food Science & Technology*, 37: 727–739.

Malouf R., Grimley Evans J. (2003) The effect of vitamin B_6 on cognition. *Cochrane Database System Revue*. (4): CD004393.

Masrizal M.A., Giraud D.W., Driskell J.A. (1997) Retention of vitamin C, iron, and beta-carotene in vegetables prepared using different cooking methods. *Journal of Food Quality*, 20(5): 403–418.

McArdle F., Rhodes L.E., Parslew R., Jack C.I., Friedmann P.S., Jackson M.J. (2002) UVR-induced oxidative stress in human skin in vivo: Effects of oral vitamin C supplementation. *Free Radical Biology & Medicine*, 33(10): 1355–1362.

McCarty M.F. (2000) Prenatal high dose pyridoxine may prevent hypertension and syndrome X in-utero by protecting the fetus from excess glucocorticoid activity. *Medical Hypotheses*, 54(5): 808–813.

Minguez-Alarcón L., Chavarro J.E., Mendiola J., et al. (2017) Fatty acid intake in relation to reproductive hormones and testicular volume among young healthy men. *Asian Journal of Andrology*, 19(2): 184–190.

Molloy A.M., Kirke P.N., Troendle J.F., et al. (2009) Maternal vitamin B_{12} status and risk of neural tube defects in a population with high neural tube defect prevalence and no folic acid fortification. *Pediatrics*, 123(3): 917–923.

Morris M.S., Picciano M.F., Jacques P.F., Selhub J. (2008) Plasma pyridoxal 5'-phosphate in the US population: The National Health and Nutrition Examination Survey, 2003–2004. *American Journal of Clinical Nutrition*, 87(5): 1446–1454.

National Institutes of Health: Office of Dietary Supplements (2019) Calcium: Fact Sheet for Health Professionals. Retrieved from ods.od.nih.gov/factsheets/Calcium-HealthProfessional/ November 23 2019.

National Institutes of Health: Office of Dietary Supplements (2019) Folate: Fact Sheet for Health Professionals. Retrieved from ods. od.nih.gov/factsheets/Folate-HealthProfessional/ November 6, 2019.

National Institutes of Health: Office of Dietary Supplements (2019) Iron: Fact Sheet for Health Professionals. Retrieved from ods. od.nih.gov/factsheets/Iron-HealthProfessional/ November 23, 2019.

National Institutes of Health: Office of Dietary Supplements (2019) Magnesium: Fact Sheet for Health Professionals. Retrieved from ods.od.nih.gov/factsheets/Magnesium-HealthProfessional/#h2 November 22, 2019.

National Institutes of Health: Office of Dietary Supplements. (2019) Nutrient Recommendations: Dietary Reference Intakes (DRI). Retrieved from ods.od.nih.gov/Health_Information/Dietary_ Reference_Intakes.aspx November 6, 2019.

National Institutes of Health: Office of Dietary Supplements (2019) Omega-3 Fatty Acids: Fact Sheet for Consumers. Retrieved from ods.od.nih.gov/factsheets/Omega3FattyAcids-Consumer/ November 23, 2019.

National Institutes of Health: Office of Dietary Supplements (2019) Potassium: Fact Sheet for Consumers. Retrieved from ods. od.nih.gov/factsheets/Potassium-HealthProfessional/ November 24, 2019.

National Institutes of Health: Office of Dietary Supplements (2019) Selenium: Fact Sheet for Health Professionals. Retrieved from ods.od.nih.gov/factsheets/Selenium-HealthProfessional/ November 22, 2019.

National Institutes of Health: Office of Dietary Supplements (2019) Vitamin A: Fact Sheet for Health Professionals. Retrieved from ods.od.nih.gov/factsheets/VitaminA-HealthProfessional/ November 23, 2019.

National Institutes of Health: Office of Dietary Supplements (2019) Vitamin B_{12}: Fact Sheet for Health Professionals. Retrieved from ods.od.nih.gov/factsheets/VitaminB$_{12}$-HealthProfessional/ November 6, 2019.

National Institutes of Health: Office of Dietary Supplements (2019) Vitamin B_6: Fact Sheet for Health Professionals. Retrieved from ods.od.nih.gov/factsheets/VitaminB$_6$-HealthProfessional/ November 22, 2019.

National Institutes of Health: Office of Dietary Supplements (2019) Vitamin C: Fact Sheet for Health Professionals. Retrieved from ods.od.nih.gov/factsheets/VitaminC-HealthProfessional/ November 24, 2019.

National Institutes of Health: Office of Dietary Supplements (2019) Vitamin D: Fact Sheet for Health Professionals. Retrieved from ods.od.nih.gov/factsheets/VitaminD-HealthProfessional/ November 23, 2019.

National Institutes of Health: Office of Dietary Supplements (2019) Zinc: Fact Sheet for Health Professionals. Retrieved from ods. od.nih.gov/factsheets/Zinc-Consumer/ November 22, 2019.

Nehra D., Lee H.D., Fallon E.M., et al. (2012) Prolonging the female reproductive lifespan and improving egg quality with dietary omega-3 fatty acids. *Aging Cell*, 11(6): 1046–1054.

Obeid R., Holzgreve W., Pietrzik K. (2019) Folate supplementation for prevention of congenital heart defects and low birth weight: An update. *Cardiovascular Diagnosis and Therapy*, 9 (Suppl 2): S424–S433.

Ottaway P.B. (1993) Stability of vitamins in food. In: Ottaway P.B. (Ed) *The Technology of Vitamins in Food*. Springer, Boston, MA.

Prasad A.S., Mantzoros C.S., Beck F.W., Hess J.W., Brewer G.J. (1996) Zinc status and serum testosterone levels of healthy adults. *Nutrition*, 12(5): 344–348.

Raigani M., Yaghmaei B., Amirjannti N., et al. (2014) The micronutrient supplements, zinc sulphate and folic acid, did not ameliorate sperm functional parameters in oligoasthenoteratozoospermic men. *Andrologia*, 46(9): 956–962.

Raloff J. (1997) The cost of too little magnesium. *Science News*, 151(18): 279.

Rink L., Gabriel P. (2000) Zinc and the immune system. *The Proceedings of the Nutrition Society*, 59: 541–552.

Rodriguez-Moran M., Simental Mendia L.E., Zambrano Galvan G., Guerrero-Romero F. (2011) The role of magnesium in type 2 diabetes: A brief based-clinical review. *Magnesium Research*, 24: 156–162.

Roffman J.L. (2018) Neuroprotective effects of prenatal folic acid supplementation: Why timing matters. *Journal of the American Medical Association: Psychiatry*, 75: 747–748.

Ronnenberg A.G., Venner S.A., Xu Z., et al. (2007) Preconception B-vitamin and homocysteine status, conception and early pregnancy loss. *American Journal of Epidemiology*, 166(3): 304–312.

Rude R.K., Singer F.R., Gruber H.E. (2009) Skeletal and hormonal effects of magnesium deficiency. *Journal of the American College of Nutrition*, 28: 131–141.

Sandstrom B. (1997) Bioavailability of zinc. *European Journal of Clinical Nutrition*, 51(1 Suppl): S17–S19.

Saunders A., Davis B.C., Garg M.L. (2013) Omega 3 polyunsaturated fatty acids and vegetarian diets. *The Medical Journal of Australia*, 199(4): S22–S26.

Scandhan K.P., Mazumdar B.N. (1981) Correlation of sodium and potassium in human seminal plasma with fertilizing capacity of normal and infertile subjects. *Andrologia*, 13(2): 147–154.

Sharma S., Litonjua A. (2014) Asthma, allergy and responses to methyl donor supplements and nutrients. *The Journal of Allergy and Clinical Immunology*, 133(5): 1246–1254.

Shipton M.J., Thachil J. (2015) Vitamin B_{12} deficiency- a 21st century perspective. *Clinical Medicine (London)*, 15(2): 145–150.

Shukla A., Rasik A.M., Patnaik G.K. (1997) Depletion of reduced glutathione, ascorbic acid, vitamin E and antioxidant defense enzymes in a healing cutaneous wound. *Free Radical Research*, 26(2): 93–101.

Siegenberg D., Baynes R.D., Bothwell T.H., et al. (1991) Ascorbic acid prevents the dose dependent inhibitory effects of polyphenols and phytates on nonheme-iron absorption. *American Journal of Clinical Nutrition*, 53: 537–541.

Simopoulos A.T.P., Leaf A., Salem N. (1999) Essentiality of and recommended dietary intakes for omega-6 and omega-3 fatty acids. *Annals of Nutrition & Metabolism*, 43: 127–130.

Sklan D. (1987) Vitamin A in human nutrition. *Progress in Food and Nutrition Science*, 1(1): 39–55.

Steinhardt R.A., Epel D., Carroll E.J., Yanagimachi, R. (1974) Is calcium ionophore a universal activator for unfertilised eggs? *Nature*, 252(5478): 41–43.

Stephanou A., Ross R., Handwerger S. (1994) Regulation of human placental lactogen expression by 1,25-dihydroxyvitamin D3. *Endocrinology*, 135(6): 2651–2656.

Stone M.S., Martyn L., Weaver C.M. (2016) Potassium intake, bioavailability, hypertension, and glucose control. *Nutrients*, 8(7): E444.

Taylor C.L., Patterson K.Y., Roseland J.M., et al., (2014) Including food 25-hydroxyvitamin D in intake estimates may reduce the discrepancy between dietary and serum measures of vitamin D status. *Journal of Nutrition*, 144: 654–659.

Tian X., Diaz F.J. (2013) Acute dietary zinc deficiency before conception compromises oocyte epigenetic programming and disrupts embryonic development. *Developmental Biology*, 376(1): 51–61.

Tucker K.L. (2009) Osteoporosis prevention and nutrition. *Current Osteoporosis Reports*, 7:111–117.

Tuntipopipat S., Zeder C., Siriprapa P., Charoenkiatkul S. (2009) Inhibitory effects of spices and herbs on iron availability. *International Journal of Food Sciences and Nutrition*, 60(1): 43–45.

United States Food and Drug Administration. (2019) CFR—Code for Federal Regulations Title 21. Retrieved from www.accessdata.fda.gov/scripts/cdrh/cfdocs/cfcfr/CFRSearch.cfm?fr=101.54 November 6, 2019.

Uriu-Adams J.Y., Keen C.L. (2010) Zinc and reproduction: Effects of zinc deficiency on prenatal and early postnatal development. *Birth Defects Research Part B*, 89: 313–325.

Valsa J., Skandhan K.P., Khan P.S., Sumangala B., Gondalia M. (2012) Split ejaculation study: Semen parameters and calcium and magnesium in seminal plasma. *Central European Journal of Urology*, 65(4): 216–218.

Weaver C.M. (1992) Calcium bioavailability and its relation to osteoporosis. *Proceedings of the Society of Experimental Biology and Medicine*, 200(2): 157–160.

Wegumuller R., Tay F., Zeder C., Brnic M., Hurrell R.F. (2014) Zinc absorption by young adults from supplemental zinc citrate is comparable with that from zinc gluconate and higher than from zinc oxide. *The Journal of Nutrition*, 144(2): 132–136.

Whelton P.K., He J. (2014) Health effects of sodium and potassium in humans. *Current Opinion in Lipidology*, 25: 75–79.

Wise A. (1995) Phytate and zinc bioavailability. *International Journal of Food Sciences and Nutrition*, 46: 53–63.

Wolf W.R., Goldschmidt R.J. (2007) Updated estimates of the selenomethionine content of NIST wheat reference materials by GC-IDMS. *Analytical and Bioanalytical Chemistry*, 387: 2449–2452.

Wong C.P., Rinaldi N.A., Ho E. (2015) Zinc deficiency enhanced inflammatory response by increasing immune cell activation and inducing IL6 promoter demethylation. *Molecular Nutrition & Food Research*, 59(5): 991–999.

Wong W.Y., Merkus H.M., Thomas C.M. (2002) Effects of folic acid and zinc sulfate on male factor subfertility: A double-blind, randomized, placebo-controlled trial. *Fertility and Sterility*, 77: 491–498.

World Health Organization. (2019) Micronutrient Deficiencies. Retrieved from www.who.int/nutrition/topics/vad/en/ November 24, 2019.

World Health Organization. (2019) Periconceptional Folic Acid Supplementation to Prevent Neural Tube Defects. Retrieved from www.who.int/elena/titles/folate_periconceptional/en/ November 6, 2019.

Zareba P., Colaci D.S., Afeiche M., et al. (2013) Semen quality in relation to antioxidant intake in a healthy male population. *Fertility and Sterility*, 100(6): 1572–1579.

Zijp I.M., Korver O., Tijburg L.B. (2000) Effect of tea and other dietary factors on iron absorption. *Critical Reviews in Food Science and Nutrition*, 40(5): 371–398.

Zile M.H. (2001) Function of vitamin A in vertebrate embryonic development. *Journal of Nutrition*, 131(3): 703–708.

Chapter 4: The Psychology of Eating Behaviors

Adriaanse M.A., Gollwitzer P.M., De Ridder D.T.M., de Witt J.B.F., Kroese F.M. (2011) Breaking habits with implementation intentions: A test of underlying processes. *Personality and Social Psychology Bulletin*, 37(4): 501–513.

Anton S.D., Gallagher J., Carey V.J., et al. (2012) Diet type and changes in food cravings following weight loss: Findings from the POUNDS LOST trial. *Eating and Weight Disorders*, 17(2): e101–e108.

Avena N.M., Bocarsly M.E., Hoebel B.G. (2012) Animal models of sugar and fat bingeing: Relationship to food addiction and increased body weight. *Methods in Molecular Biology*, 829: 351–365.

Avena N.M., Rada P., Hoebel B.G. (2008) Evidence for sugar addiction: Behavioral and neurochemical effects of intermittent, excessive sugar intake. *Neuroscience & Biobehavioral Reviews*, 32(1): 20–39.

Chao A., Grilo C.M., White M.A., Sinha R. (2015) Food cravings mediate the relationship between chronic stress and body mass index. *Journal of Health Psychology*, 20(6): 721–729.

Chavarro J.E., Rich-Edwards J.W., Rosner B.A., Willett W.C. (2006) Iron intake and risk of ovulatory infertility. *Obstetrics & Gynecology*, 108(5): 1145–1152.

Gaskins A.J. and Chavarro J.E. (2018) Diet and fertility: A review. *American Journal of Obstetrics and Gynecology*, 218(4): 379–389.

Gordon E.L., Ariel-Donges A.H., Bauman V., Merlo L.J. (2018) What is the evidence for "food addiction"? A systematic review. *Nutrients*, 10(4): 447.

Greer S.M., Goldstein A.N., Walker M.P. (2013) The impact of sleep deprivation on food desire in the human brain. *Nature Communications*, 4: 2259.

Hall K.D., Ayuketah A., Brychta R., et al. (2019) Ultra-processed diets cause excess calorie intake and weight gain: An inpatient randomized controlled trial of *ad libitum* food intake. *Cell Metabolism*, 30(1): 67–77.

Khanna P., Chattu V.K., Aeri B.T. (2019) Nutritional aspects of depression in adolescents—a systematic review. *International Journal of Preventative Medicine*, 10: 42.

Kim H.F., Ghazizadeh A., Hikosaka O. (2016) Dopamine neurons encoding long-term memory of object value for habitual behavior. *Cell*, 163(5): 1165–1175.

Koster E.P., Mojet J. (2015) From mood to food and from food to mood: A psychological perspective on the measurement of food-related emotions in consumer research. *Food Research International*, 76(2): 180–191.

Lemstra M., Yelena B., Nwankwo C., Rogers M., Moraros J. (2016) Weight loss intervention adherence and factors promoting adherence: A meta-analysis study. *Patient Preference and Adherence*, 10: 1547–1559.

Mujcic R., Oswald A.J. (2016) Evolution of well-being and happiness after increases in consumption of fruit and vegetables. *American Journal of Public Health*, 106(8): 1504–1510.

National Institutes of Health. (2012) Breaking bad habits. Retrieved from newsinhealth.nih.gov/2012/01/breaking-bad-habits November 10, 2019.

Palomba S., Daolio J., Romeo S., Battaglia F.A., Marci R., La Sala G.B. (2018) Lifestyle and fertility: The influence of stress and quality of life on female fertility. *Reproductive Biology and Endocrinology*, 16: 113.

Parylak S.L., Koob G.F., Zorrilla E.P. (2012) The dark side of food addiction. *Physiology & Behavior*, 104(1): 149–156.

Pelchat M.L., Johnson A., Chan R., Valdez J., Ragland J.D. (2004) Images of desire: Food-craving activation during fMRI. *NeuroImage*, 23(4): 1486–1493.

Schreiber L.R.N., Odlaug B.L., Grant J.E. (2013) The overlap between binge eating disorder and substance use disorders: Diagnosis and neurobiology. *Journal of Behavioral Addictions*, 2(4): 191–198.

Shell A.G., Firmin M.W. (2017) Binge eating disorder and substance use disorder: A case for food addiction. *Psychological Studies*, 62(4): 370–376.

Ulrich-Lai Y.M. (2017) Self-medication with sucrose. *Current Opinion in Behavioral Sciences*, 9: 78–83.

Vitale S.G., La Rosa V.L., Petrosino B., Rodolico A., Mineo L., Lagana A.S. (2017) The impact of lifestyle, diet, and psychological stress on female fertility. *Oman Medical Journal*, 32(5): 443–444.

Volkow N.D., Wang G.J., Baler R.D. (2012) Reward, dopamine and the control of food intake: Implications for obesity. *Trends in Cognitive Sciences*, 15(1): 37–46.

Wahl D.R., Villinger K., Konig L.M., Ziesemer K., Schupp H.T., Renner B. (2017) Healthy food choices are happy choices: Evidence from a real life sample using smartphone based assessments. *Scientific Reports*, 7: 17069.

Wiss D.A., Avena N.M., Rada P. (2018) Sugar addiction: From evolution to revolution. *Frontiers in Psychiatry*, 9: 545.

Yang C., Schnepp J., Tucker R.M. (2019) Increased hunger, food cravings, food reward and portion size selection after sleep curtailment in women without obesity. *Nutrients*, 11(3): 663.

Yaribeygi H., Panahi Y., Sahraei H., Johnston T.P., Sahebkar A. (2017) The impact of stress on body function: A review. *EXCLI Journal*, 16: 1057–1072.

Zellner D.A., Loaiza A., Gonzalez Z., et al. (2006) Food selection changes under stress. *Physiology & Behavior*, 87(4): 789–793.

Chapter 5: Twenty Foods You Should Eat to Boost Your Fertility

Afeiche M.C., Chiu Y.H., Gaskins A.J., et al. (2016) Dairy intake in relation to in vitro fertilization outcomes among women from a fertility clinic. *Human Reproduction*, 31(3): 563–571.

Afeiche M.C., Gaskins A.J., Williams P.L., et al. (2014) Processed meat intake is unfavorably and fish intake favorably associated with semen quality indicators among men attending a fertility clinic. *Journal of Nutrition*, 144(7): 1091–1098.

Assinder S., Davis R., Fenwick M., Glover A. (2007) Adult only exposure of male rats to a diet of high phytoestrogen content increases apoptosis of meiotic and post-meiotic germ cells. *Society for Reproduction and Fertility*, 133(1): 11–19.

Braga D.P., Halpern G., Setti A.S., Figueira R.C., Iaconelli A., Jr, Borges E., Jr. (2015) The impact of food intake and social habits on embryo quality and the likelihood of blastocyst formation. *Reproductive Biomedicine Online*, 31: 30–38.

Castro-Acosta M.L., Lenihan-Geels G.N., Corpe C.P., Hall W.L. (2016) Berries and anthocyanins: Promising functional food ingredients with postprandial glycaemia-lowering effects. *The Proceedings of the Nutrition Society*, 75(3): 342–355.

Centers for Disease Control and Prevention. (2010) CDC Grand Rounds: Additional opportunities to prevent neural tube defects with folic acid fortification. *MMWR Morbidity and Mortality Weekly Report*, 59(31): 980–984.

Chavarro J.E., Minguez-Alarcon L., Chiu Y.H., et al. (2016) Soy intake modifies the relation between urinary bisphenol A concentrations and pregnancy outcomes among women undergoing assisted reproduction. *The Journal of Clinical Endocrinology and Metabolism*, 101(3): 1082–1090.

Chavarro J.E., Rich-Edwards J.W., Rosner B., Willett W.C. (2007) A prospective study of dairy foods intake and anovulatory infertility. *Human Reproduction*, 22(5): 1340–1347.

Colagar A.H., Marzony E.T., Chaichi M.J. (2009) Zinc levels in seminal plasma are associated with sperm quality in fertile and infertile men. *Nutrition Research*, 29(2): 82–88.

Colpo E., Vilanova C.D., Brenner Reetz L.G., et al. (2013) A single consumption of high amounts of the Brazil nuts improves lipid profile of healthy volunteers. *Journal of Nutrition and Metabolism*, 2013: 653185.

Combs G.F., Combs S.B. (1986) The Role of Selenium in Nutrition. Academic Press; Orlando, FL, USA.

Comerford K.B., Ayoob K.T., Murray R.D., Atkinson S.A. (2016) The role of avocados in maternal diets during the periconceptional period, pregnancy, and lactation. *Nutrients*, 8(5): e313.

Coronel J., Pinos I., Amengual J. (2019) beta-carotene in obesity research: Technical considerations and current status of the field. *Nutrients*, 11(4): e842.

Cunnane S.C., Anderson M.J. (1997) The majority of dietary linoleate in growing rats is beta-oxidized or stored in visceral fat. *Journal of Nutrition*, 127:146–152.

Deepa, N., Kaur C., Singh B., Kapoor H.C. (2006) Antioxidant activity in some red sweet pepper cultivars. *Journal of Food Composition and Analysis*, 19(6–7): 572–578.

Desmewati D., Sulastri D. (2019) Phytoestrogens and their health effect. *Open Access Macedonian Journal of Medical Sciences*, 7(3): 495–499.

Djujic I.S., Jozanov-Stankov O.N., Milovac M., Jankovic V., Djermanovic V. (2000) Bioavailability and possible benefits of wheat intake naturally enriched with selenium and its products. *Biological Trace Element Research*, 77(3): 273–285.

Drouillet P., Kaminski M., Lauzon-Guillain B.D., et al. (2009) Association between maternal seafood consumption before pregnancy and fetal growth: Evidence for an association in overweight women. The EDEN Mother-child cohort. *Paediatric and Perinatal Epidemiology*, 23(1): 76–86.

Durairajanayagam D., Agarwal A., Ong C., Prashast P. (2014) Lycopene and male infertility. *Asian Journal of Andrology*, 16: 420–425.

Environmental Working Group. (2019) EWG shopper's guide to pesticides in produce. Retrieved from www.ewg.org/foodnews/summary.php#clean-fifteen December 1, 2019.

Fedder M.D., Jakobsen H.B., Giversen I., Christensen L.P., Parner E.T., Fedder J. (2014) An extract of pomegranate fruit and galangal rhizome increases the numbers of motile sperm: A prospective, randomised, controlled, double-blinded trial. *PLoS One*, 9(9): e108532.

Ferretti G., Bacchetti T., Belleggia A., Neri D. (2010) Cherry antioxidants: From farm to table. *Molecules*, 15(10): 6993–7005.

Fontana R., Della Torre S. (2016) The deep correlation between energy metabolism and reproduction: A view on the effects of nutrition for women's fertility. *Nutrients*, 8(2): 87.

Ganesan K., Xu B. (2017) Polyphenol-rich dry common beans (Phaseolus vulgaris L.) and their health benefits. *International Journal of Molecular Sciences*, 18(11): e2331.

Ganesan K., Xu B. (2017) Polyphenol-rich lentils and their health promoting effects. *International Journal of Molecular Sciences*, 18(11): e2390.

Gaskins A.J., Chavarro J.E. (2018) Diet and fertility: A review. *American Journal of Obstetrics and Gynecology*, 218(4): 379–389.

Gaskins A.J., Chiu Y-H., Williams P.L., et al. (2016) Maternal whole grain intake and outcomes of in vitro fertilization. *Fertility and Sterility*, 105(6): 1503–1510.

Gaskins A.J., Sundaram R., Buck Louis G.M., Chavarro J.E. (2018) Seafood intake, sexual activity, and time to pregnancy. *The Journal of Clinical Endocrinology and Metabolism*, 103(7): 2680–2688.

Goyal A., Chopra M., Lwaleed B.A., Birch B., Cooper A.J. (2007) The effects of dietary lycopene supplementation on human seminal plasma. *BJU International*, 99(6): 1456–1460.

Graham T.W., Thurmond M.C., Gershwin M.E., Picanso J.P., Garvey J.S., Keen C.L. (1994) Serum zinc and copper concentrations in relation to spontaneous abortion to cows: Implications for human fetal loss. *Journal of Reproduction and Fertility*, 102: 253–262.

Grieger J.A., Grzeskowiak L.E., Wilson R.L., et al. (2019) Maternal selenium, copper and zinc concentrations in early pregnancy, and the association with fertility. *Nutrients*, 11(7): e1609.

Gupta R.K., Gangoliya S.S., Singh N.K. (2015) Reduction of phytic acid and enhancement of bioavailable micronutrients in food grains. *Journal of Food Science and Technology*, 52(2): 676–684.

Hamilton M.C., Hites R.A., Schwager S.J., Foran J.A., Knuth B.A., Carpenter D.O. (2005) Lipid composition and contaminants in farmed and wild salmon. *Environmental Science and Technology*, 39(22): 8622–8629.

Hasler C.M. (1998) Functional foods: Their role in disease prevention and health. *Food Technology*, 52: 63–69.

Hemken R.W., Bremel D.H. (1982) Possible role of beta-carotene in improving fertility in dairy cattle. *Journal of Dairy Science*, 65(7): 1069–1073.

Howe J.C. (1990) Postprandial response of calcium metabolism in postmenopausal women to meals varying in protein level/ source. *Metabolism*, 39: 1246–1252.

Iammarino M., Di Taranto A., Cristino M. (2014) Monitoring of nitrites and nitrate levels in leafy vegetables (spinach and lettuce): A contribution to risk assessment. *Journal of the Science of Food and Agriculture*, 15: 773–778.

Jin H., Zhang Y.J., Jiang J.X., et al. (2013) Studies on the extraction of pumpkin components and their biological effects on blood glucose of diabetic mice. *Journal of Food Drug Analysis*, 21: 184–189.

Jenkins D.J.A., Kendall C.W.C., Vidgen E., et al. (1999) Health aspects of partially defatted flaxseed, including effects on serum lipids, oxidative measures, and ex vivo androgen and progestin activity: A controlled crossover trial. *American Journal of Clinical Nutrition*, 69: 395–402.

Kaulmann A., Legay S., Schneider Y.J., Hoffmann L., Bohn T. (2016) Inflammation related responses of intestinal cells to plum and cabbage digesta with differential carotenoid and polyphenol profiles following simulated gastrointestinal digestion. *Molecular Nutrition and Food Research*, 60(5): 992–1005.

Kelkitli E., Ozturk N., Aslan N.A., et al. (2016) Serum zinc levels in patients with iron deficiency anemia and its association with symptoms of iron deficiency anemia. *Annals of Hematology*, 95(5): 751–756.

Kim K., Schisterman E.F., Silver R.M., et al. (2018) Shorter time to pregnancy with increasing preconception carotene concentrations among women with 1–2 previous pregnancy losses. *American Journal of Epidemiology*, 187(9): 1907–1915.

Koss-Mikolajczyk I., Kusznierewicz B., Wiczkowski W., Platosz N., Bartoszek A. (2019) Phytochemical composition and biological activities of differently pigmented cabbage (Brassica oleracea var. capitata) and cauliflower (Brassica oleracea var. botrytis) varieties. *Journal of the Science of Food and Agriculture*, 99(12): 5499–5507.

Kris-Etherton P.M. (1999) AHA Science Advisory. Monounsaturated fatty acids and risk of cardiovascular disease. American Heart Association. Nutrition Committee. *Circulation*, 100(11): 1253–1258.

Kuiper G.G., Lemmen J.G., Carlsson B., et al. (1998) Interaction of estrogenic chemicals and phytoestrogens with estrogen receptor beta. *Endocrinology*, 139: 4252–4263.

Li Y., Yao J., Han C., et al. (2016) Quercetin, inflammation and immunity. *Nutrients*, 8(3): 167.

Ly C., Yockell-Lelievre J., Ferraro Z.M., Arnason J.T., Ferrier J., Gruslin A. (2015) The effects of dietary polyphenols on reproductive health and early development. *Human Reproduction Update*, 21(2): 228–248.

MacDougall A.J., Selvendran R.R. (2001) Chemistry, architecture, and composition of dietary fiber from plant cell walls. In *Handbook of Dietary Fiber*, pp. 281–319 (S.S. Cho and M.L. Dreher, editors). New York: Marcel Dekker, Inc.

Maeda E., Murata K., Kumazawa Y., et al. (2019) Associations of environmental exposures to methylmercury and selenium with female infertility: A case-control study. *Environmental Research*, 168: 357–363.

Matsfuji H., Ishikawa K., Nunomura O., Chino M., Takeda M. (2007) Antioxidant content of different sweet peppers, white, green, yellow, orange and red (Capsicum annuum L). *Journal of Food Science and Technology*, 42(12): 1482–1488.

Mensink R.P., Zock P.L., Kester A.D.M., Katan M.B. (2003) Effects of dietary fatty acids and carbohydrates on the ratio of serum total to HDL cholesterol and on serum lipids and apolipoproteins: A meta-analysis of 60 controlled trials. *American Journal of Clinical Nutrition*, 77(5): 1146–1155.

Minich D.M. (2019) A review of the science of colorful, plant-based food and practical strategies for "Eating the Rainbow". *Journal of Nutrition and Metabolism*, 2019: 1–19.

Moran L.J., Tsagareli V., Noakes M., Norman R. (2016) Altered preconception fatty acid intake is associated with improved pregnancy rates in overweight and obese women undertaking in vitro fertilization. *Nutrients*, 8: E10.

Mounien L., Tourniaire F., Landrier J-F. (2019) Anti-obesity effect of carotenoids: Direct impact on adipose tissue and adipose tissue-driven indirect effects. *Nutrients*, 11(7): 1562.

Mozaffarian D., Katan M.B., Ascherio A., Stampfer M.J., Willett W.C. (2006) Trans fatty acids and cardiovascular disease. *New England Journal of Medicine*, 354(15): 1601–1613.

Mozaffarian D., Rimm E.B. (2006) Fish intake, contaminants, and human health: Evaluating the risks and the benefits. *Journal of the American Medical Association*, 296: 1885–1899.

Mueller S.O. (2002) Overview of in vitro tools to assess the estrogenic and antiestrogenic activity of phytoestrogens. *Journal of Chromatography B*, 777: 155–165.

Mumford S.L., Kim S., Chen Z., Barr D.B., Louis G. (2015) Urinary phytoestrogens are associated with subtle indicators of semen quality among male partners of couples desiring pregnancy. *The Journal of Nutrition*, 145(11): 2535–2541.

Nassan F.L., Chiu Y.H., Vanegas J.C., et al. (2018) Intake of protein-rich foods in relation to outcomes of infertility treatment with assisted reproductive technologies. *American Journal of Clinical Nutrition*, 108(5): 1104–1112.

National Institutes of Health: Office of Dietary Supplements (2019) Iron: Fact Sheet for Health Professionals. Retrieved from ods.od.nih.gov/factsheets/Iron-HealthProfessional/ November 23, 2019.

National Institutes of Health: Office of Dietary Supplements (2019) Vitamin B_6: Fact Sheet for Health Professionals. Retrieved from ods.od.nih.gov/factsheets/VitaminB$_6$-HealthProfessional/ November 22, 2019.

National Institutes of Health: Office of Dietary Supplements (2019) Vitamin D: Fact Sheet for Health Professionals. Retrieved from ods.od.nih.gov/factsheets/VitaminD-HealthProfessional/ November 23, 2019.

Nehra D., Le H.D., Fallon E.M., et al. (2012) Prolonging the female reproductive lifespan and improving egg quality with dietary omega-3 fatty acids. *Aging Cell*, 11: 1046–1054.

Norman G., Hord N.G., Tang Y., Bryan N.S. (2009) Food sources of nitrates and nitrites: The physiologic context for potential health benefits. *American Journal of Clinical Nutrition*, 90(1): 1–10.

Parisi F., Rousian M., Huijgen N.A., et al. (2017) Periconceptional maternal "high fish and olive oil, low meat" dietary pattern is associated with increased embryonic growth: The Rotterdam Periconceptional Cohort (Predict) Study. *Ultrasound in Obstetrics and Gynecology*, 50(6): 709–716.

Patel S., Hartman J.A., Helferich W.G., Flaws J.A. (2017) Preconception exposure to dietary levels of genistein affects female reproductive outcomes. *Reproductive Toxicology*, 74: 174–180.

Patel S., Rauf A. (2017) Edible seeds from cucurbitaceae family as potential functional foods: Immense promises, few concerns. *Biomedicine & Pharmacotherapy*, 91: 330–337.

Patisaul H.B. (2017) Endocrine disruption by dietary phytoestrogens: Impact on dimorphic sexual systems and behaviors. *The Proceedings of the Nutrition Society*, 76(2): 130–144.

Podesedek A. (2007) Natural antioxidants and antioxidant capacity of Brassica vegetables: A review. *Food Science and Technology*. 40(1): 1–11.

Qu H., Madl R.L., Takemoto D.L., Baybutt R.C., Wang W. (2005) Lignans are involved in the antitumor activity of wheat bran in colon cancer SW480 cells. *Journal of Nutrition*, 135: 598–602.

Rao A.V., Waseem Z., Agarwal S. (1998) Lycopene content of tomatoes and tomato products and their contribution to dietary lycopene. *Food Research International*, 31(10): 737–741.

Rietjens I., Louisse J., Beekmann K. (2017) The potential health effects of dietary phytoestrogens. *British Journal of Pharmacology*, 174(11): 1263–1280.

Rudolph M.D., Graham A.M., Feczko E., et al. (2018) Maternal IL-6 during pregnancy can be estimated from newborn brain connectivity and predicts future working memory in offspring. *Nature Neuroscience*, 21: 765–772.

Scanlan R.A. (1983) Formation and occurrence of nitrosamines in food. *Cancer Research*, 43(5 Suppl): 2435s-2440s.

Sierens J., Hartley J.A., Campbell M.J., Leathem A.J., Woodside J.V. (2001) Effect of phytoestrogen and antioxidant supplementation on oxidative DNA damage assessed using the comet assay. *Mutation Research*, 485(2): 169–176.

Silva E.O., Bracarense A.P. (2016) Phytic acid: From antinutritional to multiple protection factor of organic systems. *Journal of Food Science*, 81(6): R1357–1362.

Simmer K., Thompson R.P. (1985) Maternal zinc and intrauterine growth retardation. *Clinical Science*, 68(4): 395–399.

Slavin J., Jacobs D., Marquart L. (1997) Whole-grain consumption and chronic disease: Protective mechanisms. *Nutrition and Cancer*, 27: 14–21.

Sreekumar S., Sithul H., Muraleedharan P., Azeez J.M., Sreeharshan S. (2014) Pomegranate fruit as a rich source of biologically active compounds. *BioMed Research International*, 2014: 686921.

US Food and Drug Administration. Mercury Levels in Commercial Fish and Shellfish (1990–2012). Retrieved from www.fda.gov/food/metals/mercury-levels-commercial-fish-and-shellfish-1990–2012 December 9, 2019.

Vanegas J.C., Afeiche M.C., Gaskins A.J., et al. (2015). Soy food intake and treatment outcomes of women undergoing assisted reproductive treatment. *Fertility and Sterility*, 103(3): 749–755.

Vujkovic M., de Vries J.H., Lindemans J., et al. (2010) The preconception Mediterranean dietary pattern in couples undergoing in vitro fertilization/intracytoplasmic sperm injection treatment increases the chance of pregnancy. *Fertility and Sterility*, 94(6): 2096–2101.

Wise L.A., Wesselink A.K., Tucker K.L., et al. (2018) Dietary fat intake and fecundability in 2 preconception cohort studies. *American Journal of Epidemiology*, 187(1): 60–74.

Wolk A. (2017) Potential health hazards of eating red meat. *Journal of Internal Medicine*, 281(2): 106–122.

Xanthopoulou M.N., Nomikos T., Fragopoulou E., Antonopoulou S. Antioxidant and lipoxygenase inhibitory activities of pumpkin seed extracts. *Food Research International*, 42(5–6): 641–646.

Yu S., Zhao Y., Feng Y., et al. (2019) beta-carotene improves oocyte development and maturation under oxidative stress in vitro. *In Vitro Cellular & Developmental Biology: Animal*, 55(7): 548–558.

Yuan G., Liu Y., Liu G., et al. (2019) Associations between semen phytoestrogens concentrations and semen quality in Chinese men. *Environment International*, 129: 136–144.

Zhang B., Deng Z., Tang Y., et al. (2017) Bioaccessibility, in vitro antioxidant and anti-inflammatory activities of phenolics in cooked green lentil (Lens culinaris). *Journal of Functional Foods*, 32: 248–255.

Zhang Z., Fulgoni V.L., Kris-Etherton P.M., Mitmesser S.H. (2018) Dietary intakes of EPA and DHA omega-3 fatty acids among US childbearing-age and pregnant women: An analysis of NHANES 2001–2014. *Nutrients*,10(4): 416.

Zheng Y., Li Y., Satija A., et al. (2019) Association of changes in red meat consumption with total and cause specific mortality among US women and men: Two prospective cohort studies. *BMJ*, 365: 12110

Zhou K., Su L., Yu L. (2004) Phytochemicals and antioxidant properties in wheat bran. *Journal of Agricultural and Food Chemistry*, 52: 6108–6114.

Zini A., San Gabriel M., Libman J. (2010) Lycopene supplementation in vitro can protect human sperm deoxyribonucleic acid from oxidative damage. *Fertility and Sterility*, 94(3): 1033–1036.

Chapter 6: Twenty Foods You Should Avoid (or Limit) When You Want to Get Pregnant

Adekunbi D.A., Ogunsola O.A., Oyelowo O.T., et al. (2016) Consumption of high sucrose and/or high salt diet alters sperm function in male Sprague-Dawley rats. *Egyptian Journal of Basic and Applied Sciences*, 3(2): 194–201.

American Heart Association (2018) Added sugars. Retrieved from www.heart.org/en/healthy-living/healthy-eating/eat-smart/sugar/added-sugars December 3, 2019.

American Heart Association. (2018) Sodium sources: Where does all that sodium come from. Retrieved from www.heart.org/en/healthy-living/healthy-eating/eat-smart/sodium/sodium-sources December 3, 2019.

Antoniotti G.S., Coughlan M., Salamonsen L.A., Evans J. (2018) Obesity associated advanced glycation end products within the human uterine cavity adversely impact endometrial function and embryo implantation competence. *Human Reproduction*, 33(4): 654–665.

Aronow W.S. (2017) Reduction in dietary sodium improves blood pressure and reduces cardiovascular events and mortality. *Annals of Translational Medicine*, 5(20): 405.

Bach C.C., Vested A., Jorgensen K.T., Bonde J.P., Henriksen T.B., Toft G. (2016) Perfluoroalkyl and polyfluoroalkyl substances and measures of human fertility: A systematic review. *Critical Reviews in Toxicology*, 46(9): 735–755.

Bao W., Tobias D.K., Olsen S.F., Zhang C. (2014) Pre-pregnancy fried food consumption and the risk of gestational diabetes mellitus: A prospective cohort study. *Diabetologia*, 57(12): 2485–2491.

Bjorklund G., Chirumbolo S., Dadar M., et al. (2019) Mercury exposure and its effects on fertility and pregnancy outcome. *Basic & Clinical Pharmacology & Toxicology*, 125(4): 317–327.

Braga D.P., Halpern G., Setti A.S., Figueira R.C., Iaconelli A., Jr., Borges E., Jr. (2015) The impact of food intake and social habits on embryo quality and the likelihood of blastocyst formation. *Reproductive Biomedicine Online*, 31(1): 30–38.

Cabler S., Agarwal A., Flint M., Du Plessis S.S. (2010) Obesity: Modern man's fertility nemesis. *Asian Journal of Andrology*, 12(4): 480–489.

Chen L., Xie Y.M., Pei J.H., et al. (2018) Sugar-sweetened beverage intake and serum testosterone levels in adult males 20–39 years old in the United States. *Reproductive Biology and Endocrinology*,16(1): 61.

Ding G.L., Liu Y., Liu M.E., et al. (2015) The effects of diabetes on male fertility and epigenetic regulation during spermatogenesis. *Asian Journal of Andrology*, 17(6): 948–953.

Duan X., Wang Q.C., Chen K.L., Zhu C.C., Liu J., Sun S.C. (2015) Acrylamide toxic effects on mouse oocyte quality and fertility in vivo. *Scientific Reports*, 5: 11562.

Efrat M.E., Stein A., Pinkas H., Unger R., Birk R. (2018) Dietary patterns are positively associated with semen quality. *Fertility and Sterility*, 109(5): 809–816.

Ehrlich S., Williams P.L., Missmer S.A., et al. (2012) Urinary bisphenol A concentrations and early reproductive health outcomes among women undergoing IVF. *Human Reproduction*, 27(12): 3583–3592.

Elewa Y.H.A., Mohamed A.A., Galal A.A.A., El-Naseery N.I., Ichii O., Kon Y. (2019) Food Yellow4 reprotoxicity in relation to localization of DMC1 and apoptosis in rat testes: Roles of royal jelly and cod liver oil. *Ecotoxicology and Environmental Safety*, 169: 696–706.

Eweka A.O., Om'Iniabohs F.A.E. (2011) Histological studies of the effects of monosodium glutamate on the ovaries of adult Wistar rats. *Annals of Medical and Health Sciences Research*, 1(1): 37–43.

Fallah A., Mohammad-Hasani A., Colagar A.H. (2018) Zinc is an essential element for male fertility: A review of Zn roles in men's health, germination, sperm quality and fertilization. *Journal of Reproduction & Infertility*, 19(2): 69–81.

Fontana R., Della Torre S. (2016) The deep correlation between energy metabolism and reproduction: A view on the effects of nutrition for women's fertility. *Nutrients*, 8(2): 87.

Franck U., Weller A., Roder S.W., et al. (2014) Prenatal VOC exposure and redecoration are related to wheezing in early infancy. *Environment International*, 73: 393–401.

Gaskins A.J., Chavarro J.E. (2018) Diet and fertility: A review. *American Journal of Obstetrics and Gynecology*, 218(4): 379–389.

Gaskins A.J., Nassan F.L., Chiu Y-H., et al. (2019) Dietary patterns and outcomes of assisted reproduction. *American Journal of Obstetrics and Gynecology*, 220(6): 567.e561–567.e518.

Gelbke H.P., Banton M., Block C., et al. (2018) Oligomers of styrene are not endocrine disruptors. *Critical Reviews in Toxicology*, 48(6): 471–499.

Ghosh I., Sharma P.K., Rahman M., Lahkar K. (2019) Sugar-sweetened beverage intake in relation to semen quality in infertile couples: A prospective observational study. *Fertility Science and Research*, 6(1): 40–48.

Gray C., Long S., Green C., et al. (2013). Maternal fructose and/or salt intake and reproductive outcome in the rat: Effects on growth, fertility, sex ratio, and birth order. *Biology of Reproduction*, 89(3): 1–8.

Grieger J.A., Grzeskowiak L.E., Bianco-Miotto T., et al. (2018) Pre-pregnancy fast food and fruit intake is associated with time to pregnancy. *Human Reproduction*, 33(6): 1063–1070.

Halpern G., Braga D.P., Setti A.S., Figueira R.C., Iaconelli Jr. A., Borges Jr E. (2016) Artificial sweeteners: Do they bear an infertility risk? *Fertility and Sterility*, 106(3): e263.

Hatch E.E., Wesselink A.K., Hahn K.A., et al. (2018). Intake of sugar-sweetened beverages and fecundability in a North American preconception cohort. *Epidemiology*, 29(3): 369–378.

Hartle J.C., Navas-Acien A., Lawrence R.S. (2016) The consumption of canned food and beverages and urinary Bisphenol A concentrations in NHANES 2003–2008. *Environmental Research*, 150: 375–382.

Hohos N.M., Cho K.J., Swindle D.C., Skaznik-Wikiel M.E. (2018) High-fat diet exposure, regardless of induction of obesity, is associated with altered expression of genes critical to normal ovulatory function. *Molecular and Cellular Endocrinology*, 470: 199–207.

Kadawathagedara M., Botton J., de Lauzon-Guillain B., et al. (2018) Dietary acrylamide intake during pregnancy and postnatal growth and obesity: Results from the Norwegian Mother and Child Cohort Study (MoBa). *Environment International*, 113: 325–334.

Kobylewski S., Jacobson M.F. (2012) Toxicology of food dyes. *International Journal of Occupational and Environmental Health*,18(3): 220–246.

Li P., Hua R., Li K., et al. (2018) Polycyclic aromatic hydrocarbons exposure and early miscarriage in women undergoing in vitro fertilization-embryo transfer. *Human Fertility*, 1–6.

Livshits A., Seidman D.S. (2009) Fertility issues in women with diabetes. *Women's Health*, 5(6): 701–707.

Lyngso J., Ramlau-Hansen C.H., Bay B., Ingerslev H.J., Strandberg-Larsen K., Kesmodel U.S. (2019) Low-to-moderate alcohol consumption and success in fertility treatment: A Danish cohort study. *Human Reproduction*, 34(7): 1334–1344.

Machtinger R., Combelles C.M.H., Missmer S.A., et al. (2013) Bisphenol-A and human oocyte maturation in vitro. *Human Reproduction*, 28(10): 2735–2745.

Maeda E., Murata K., Kumazawa Y., et al. (2019) Associations of environmental exposures to methylmercury and selenium with female infertility: A case-control study. *Environmental Research*, 168: 357–363.

Malik V.S., Li Y., Pan A., et al. (2019) Long-term consumption of sugar-sweetened and artificially sweetened beverages and risk of mortality in US adults. *Circulation*, 139(18): 2113–2125.

Matuszczak E., Komarowska M.D., Debek W., Hermanowicz A. (2019) The impact of Bisphenol A on fertility, reproductive system, and development: A review of the literature. *International Journal of Endocrinology*, 2019: 4068717.

Mohammadyan M., Moosazadeh M., Borji A., Khanjani N., Rahimi Moghadam S., Behjati Moghadam A.M. (2019) Health risk assessment of occupational exposure to styrene in Neyshabur electronic industries. *Environmental Science and Pollution Research International*, 26(12): 11920–11927.

Nassan F.L., Chiu Y.H., Vanegas J.C., et al. (2018) Intake of protein-rich foods in relation to outcomes of infertility treatment with assisted reproductive technologies. *American Journal of Clinical Nutrition*,108(5): 1104–1112.

Oostingh E.C., Hall J., Koster M.P.H., Grace B., Jauniaux E., Steegers-Theunissen R.P.M. (2019) The impact of maternal lifestyle factors on periconception outcomes: A systematic review of observational studies. *Reproductive Biomedicine Online*, 38(1): 77–94.

Panth N., Gavarkovs A., Tamez M., Mattei J. (2018) The influence of diet on fertility and the implications for public health nutrition in the United States. *Frontiers in Public Health*, 6: 211.

Parisi F., Rousian M., Huijgen N.A., et al. (2017) Periconceptional maternal 'high fish and olive oil, low meat' dietary pattern is associated with increased embryonic growth: The Rotterdam Periconceptional Cohort (Predict) Study. *Ultrasound in Obstetrics and Gynecology*, 50(6): 709–716.

Pearlman M., Obert J., Casey L. (2017) The association between artificial sweeteners and obesity. *Current Gastroenterology Reports*, 19(12): 64.

Rattan S., Zhou C., Chiang C., et al. (2017) Exposure to endocrine disruptors during adulthood: Consequences for female fertility. *The Journal of Endocrinology*, 233(3): R109–R129.

Rickman J.C., Barrett D.M., Bruhn C.M. (2007) Nutritional comparison of fresh, frozen and canned fruits and vegetables. Part 1. Vitamins C and B and phenolic compounds. *Journal of the Science of Food and Agriculture*, 87(6): 930–944.

Rochester J.R., Bolden A.L. (2015) Bisphenol S and F: A systematic review and comparison of the hormonal activity of Bisphenol A substitutes. *Environmental Health Perspectives*, 123(7): 643–650.

Salas-Huetos A., Bullo M., Salas-Salvado J. (2017) Dietary patterns, foods and nutrients in male fertility parameters and fecundability: A systematic review of observational studies. *Human Reproduction Update*, 23(4): 371–389.

Sedes L., Desdoits-Lethimonier C., Rouaisnel B., et al. (2018) Crosstalk between BPA and FXRa signaling pathways lead to alterations of undifferentiated germ cell homeostasis and male fertility disorders. *Stem Cell Reports*, 11(4): 944–958.

Setti A.S., Braga D., Halpern G., Figueira R.C.S., Iaconelli A., Jr., Borges E., Jr. (2018) Is there an association between artificial sweetener consumption and assisted reproduction outcomes? *Reproductive Biomedicine Online*, 36(2): 145–153.

Shreenath A.P., Dooley J. (2019) Selenium Deficiency. StatPearls Publishing. Retrieved from www.ncbi.nlm.nih.gov/books/NBK482260/ December 5, 2019.

Silva T., Jesus M., Cagigal C., Silva C. (2019) Food with influence in sexual and reproductive health. *Current Pharmaceutical Biotechnology*, 20(2): 114–122.

Silvestris E., Lovero D., Palmirotta R. (2019) Nutrition and female fertility: An independent correlation. *Frontiers in Endocrinology*, 10: 346.

Sylvetsky A.C., Rother K.I. (2018) Nonnutritive sweeteners in weight management and chronic disease: A review. *Obesity*, 26(4): 635–640.

Uribarri J., Woodruff S., Goodman S., et al. (2010) Advanced glycation end products in foods and a practical guide to their reduction in the diet. *Journal of the American Dietetic Association*, 110(6): 911–916.

US Environmental Protection Agency. (2019) Health Effects of Exposures to Mercury. Retrieved from www.epa.gov/mercury/health-effects-exposures-mercury December 5, 2019.

US Food and Drug Administration. (2014) Bisphenol A (BPA): Use in food contact application, FDA. Retrieved from www.fda.gov/food/food-additives-petitions/bisphenol-bpa-use-food-contact-application#summary December 3, 2019.

Wang G., Yeung C.K., Zhang J.L., et al. (2015) High salt intake negatively impacts ovarian follicle development. *Annals of Anatomy—Anatomisher Anzeiger*, 200: 79–87.

Wise L.A., Wesselink A.K., Tucker K.L., et al. (2018) Dietary fat intake and fecundability in 2 preconception cohort studies. *American Journal of Epidemiology*, 187(1): 60–74.

Wolk A. (2017) Potential health hazards of eating red meat. *Journal of Internal Medicine*, 281(2): 106–122.

Zhang Z., Venn B.J., Monro J., Mishra S. (2018) Subjective satiety following meals incorporating rice, pasta and potato. *Nutrients*, 10(11): e1739.

Chapter 7: Implementing the Plan: A Guide for You and Your Partner

American Heart Association. (2017) Control your cholesterol. Retrieved from www.heart.org/en/health-topics/cholesterol/about-cholesterol December 10, 2019.

American Heart Association. (2017) Trans fats. Retrieved from www.heart.org/en/healthy-living/healthy-eating/eat-smart/fats/trans-fat December 10, 2019.

American Heart Association. (2018) Added sugars. Retrieved from www.heart.org/en/healthy-living/healthy-eating/eat-smart/sugar/added-sugars December 10, 2019.

American Heart Association. (2018) Get the scoop on sodium and salt. Retrieved from www.heart.org/en/healthy-living/healthy-eating/eat-smart/sodium/sodium-and-salt December 10, 2019.

American Heart Association. (2018) How much sodium should I eat per day? Retrieved from www.heart.org/en/healthy-living/healthy-eating/eat-smart/sodium/how-much-sodium-should-i-eat-per-day December 10, 2019.

American Heart Association. (2019) Saturated Fat. Retrieved from www.heart.org/en/healthy-living/healthy-eating/eat-smart/fats/saturated-fats December 10, 2019.

Casu G., Zaia V., Fernandes Martins Md.C., Parente Barbosa C., Gremigni P. (2019) A dyadic mediation study on social support, coping, and stress among couples starting fertility treatment. *Journal of Family Psychology*, 33(3): 315–326.

Chavarro J.E., Rich-Edwards J.W., Rosner B.A., Willett W.C. (2006) Iron intake and risk of ovulatory infertility. *Obstetrics & Gynecology*, 108(5): 1145–1152.

Gaskins A.J., Chavarro J.E. (2018) Diet and fertility: A review. *American Journal of Obstetrics and Gynecology*, 218(4): 379–389.

Hoffman J.R., Falvo M.J. (2004) Protein—which is best? *Journal of Sports Science and Medicine*, 3(3): 118–130.

Krauss R.M., Eckel R.H., Howard B., et al. (2000) AHA Dietary guidelines. *Journal of the American Heart Association*, 102: 2284–2299.

Kroemeke A., Kubicka E. (2018) Positive and negative adjustment in couples undergoing fertility treatment: The impact of support exchange. *PLOS One*, 13(6): e0200124.

Metzgar C.J., Preston A.G., Miller D.L., Nickols-Richardson S.M. (2015) Facilitators and barriers to weight loss and weight loss maintenance: A qualitative exploration. *Journal of Human Nutrition and Dietetics*, 28: 593–603.

Office of Disease Prevention and Health Promotion. (2015) Dietary Guidelines for Americans. Retrieved from health.gov/dietaryguidelines/2015/guidelines/appendix-2/ December 10, 2019.

Ozaki I., Watai I., Nishijima M., Saito N. (2018) Randomized controlled trial of web-based weight-loss intervention with human support for male workers under 40. *Journal of Occupational Health*, 61: 110–120.

The National Academies of Sciences, Engineering and Medicine. (2002) Dietary reference intakes for energy, carbohydrate, fiber, fat, fatty acids, cholesterol, protein, and amino acids, Retrieved from nationalacademies.org/hmd/~/media/Files/Activity percent20Files/Nutrition/DRI-Tables/8_Macronutrient percent20Summary.pdf December 10, 2019.

Palomba S., Daolio J., Romeo S., Battaglia F.A., Marci R., La Sala G.B. (2018) Lifestyle and fertility: The influence of stress and quality of life on female fertility. *Reproductive Biology and Endocrinology*, 16: 113.

Patel A., Sharma P.S.V.N., Kumar P., Binu V.S. (2018) Sociocultural determinants of infertility stress in patients undergoing fertility treatments. *Journal of Human Reproductive Sciences*, 11(2): 172–179.

Riebl S.K., Davy B.M. (2013) The hydration equation: Update on water balance and cognitive performance. *ACSM's Health & Fitness Journal*, 17(6): 21–28.

Schaafsma G. (2000) Protein digestibility-corrected amino acid score. *Journal of Nutrition*, 130(7): 1865S-1867S.

Vitale S.G., La Rosa V.L., Petrosino B., Rodolico A., Mineo L., Lagana A.S. (2017) The impact of lifestyle, diet, and psychological stress on female fertility. *Oman Medical Journal*, 32(5): 443–444.

Xenaki N., Bacopoulou F., Kokkinos A., Nicolaides N.C., Chrousos G.P., Darviri C. (2018) Impact of a stress management program on weight loss, mental health, and lifestyle in adults with obesity: A randomized controlled trial. *Journal of Molecular Biochemistry*, 7(2): 78–84.

Yaribeygi H., Panahi Y., Sahraei H., Johnston T.P., Sahebkar A. (2017) The impact of stress on body function: A review. *EXCLI Journal*, 16: 1057–1072.

Chapter 8: Beyond Food: What You Need to Know About Toxins

Albert O., Huang J.Y., Aleska K., et al. (2018) Exposure to polybrominated diphenyl ethers and phthalates in healthy men living in the greater Montreal area: A study of hormonal balance and semen quality. *Environmental International*, 116: 165–175.

Al-Saleh I., Coskun S., Al-Doush I., et al. (2019) Exposure to phthalates in couples undergoing in-vitro fertilization treatment and its association with oxidative stress and DNA damage. *Environmental Research*, 169: 396–408.

Bach C.C., Vested A., Jorgensen K.T., Bonde J.P., Henriksen T.B., Toft G. (2016) Perfluoroalkyl and polyfluoroalkyl substances and measures of human fertility: A systematic review. *Critical Reviews in Toxicology*, 46(9): 735–755.

Bellavia A., Chiu Y.H., Brown F.M., et al. (2019) Urinary concentrations of parabens mixture and pregnancy glucose levels among women from a fertility clinic. *Environmental Research*, 168: 389–396.

Biotechnology Innovation Organization. (2019) Genetically Engineered Animals: Frequently Asked Questions. Biotechnology Innovation Organization. Retrieved from www.bio.org/articles/genetically-engineered-animals-frequently-asked-questions November 2, 2019.

Brents L.K. (2016) Marijuana, the endocannabinoid system and the female reproductive system. *The Yale Journal of Biology and Medicine*, 89(2): 175–191.

Carvalho R.K., Andersen M.L., Mazaro-Costa R. (2019) The effects of cannabidiol on male reproductive system: A literature review. *Journal of Applied Toxicology*, [Epub ahead of print].

Center for Food Safety. (2019) About Genetically Engineered Foods. Retrieved from www.centerforfoodsafety.org/issues/311/ge-foods/about-ge-foods December 11, 2019.

Chevrier C., Warembourg C., Gaudreau E., et al. (2013) Organochlorine pesticides, polychlorinated biphenyls, seafood consumption, and time-to-pregnancy. *Epidemiology*, 24(2): 251–260.

Chiu Y.H., Williams P.L., Gillman M.W., et al. (2018) Association between pesticide residue intake from consumption of fruits and vegetables and pregnancy outcomes among women undergoing infertility treatment with assisted reproductive technology. *Journal of the American Medical Association*, 178(1): 17–26.

Collins G.G., Rossi B.V. (2015) The impact of lifestyle modifications, diet, and vitamin supplementation on natural fertility. *Fertility Research and Practice*, 1: 11.

Di Nisio A., Sabovic I., Valente U., et al. (2019) Endocrine disruption of androgenic activity by perfluoroalkyl substances: Clinical and experimental evidence. *The Journal of Clinical Endocrinology and Metabolism*, 104(4): 1259–1271.

El-Shamei Z.S., Gab-Alla A.A., Shatta A.A., Moussa E.A., Rayan A.M. (2012) Histopathological changes in some organs of male rats fed on genetically modified corn (Ajeeb YG). *Journal of American Science*, 8(10): 684–696.

Environmental Working Group. (2018) Environmental Working Group's Guide to Avoiding PFAS Chemicals. Retrieved from static.ewg.org/ewg-tip-sheets/EWG-AvoidingPFCs.pdf?_ga=2.48203491.570618924.1570831767-1623339879.1570831767 December 11, 2019.

Fujino C., Watanabe Y., Sanoh S., et al. (2019) Comparative study of the effect of 17 parabens on PXR-, CAR- and PPARalpha-mediated transcriptional activation. *Food and Chemical Toxicology*, 133: 110792.

Gab-Alla A.A., El-Shamei Z.S., Shatta A.A., Moussa E.A., Rayan A.M. (2012) Morphological and biochemical changes in male rats fed on genetically modified corn (Ajeeb YG). *Journal of American Science*, 8(9): 1117–1123.

Gao M., Li B., Wenzhen Y., Zhao L., Zhang X. (2014) Hypothetical link between infertility and genetically modified food. *Recent Patents on Food, Nutrition & Agriculture*, 6(1): 16–22.

Gao M., Yuan W., Zhao L., Zhang X. (2014) Hypothetical link between infertility and genetically modified food. *Recent Patents on Food, Nutrition & Agriculture*, 6(1): 16–22.

Gaskins A.J., Fong K.C., Abu Awad Y., et al. (2019) Time-varying exposure to air pollution and outcomes of in vitro fertilization among couples from a fertility clinic. *Environmental Health Perspectives*, 127(7): 77002.

Gaskins A.J., Minguez-Alarcon L., Fong K.C., et al. (2019) Supplemental folate and the relationship between traffic-related air pollution and livebirth among women undergoing assisted reproduction. *American Journal of Epidemiology*, 188(9): 1595–1604.

Gaskins A.J., Nassan F.L., Chiu Y-H., et al. (2019) Dietary patterns and outcomes of assisted reproduction. *American Journal of Obstetrics and Gynecology*, 220(6): 567.e561–567.e518.

Glockner G., Seralini G.E. (2016) Pathology reports on the first cows fed with Bt175 maize (1997–2002). *Scholarly Journal of Agricultural Sciences*, 6(1): 1–8.

Gunes S., Metin Mahmutoglu A., Arslan M.A., Henkel R. (2018) Smoking-induced genetic and epigenetic alterations in infertile men. *Andrologia*, 50(9): e13124.

Hauser R., Gaskins A.J., Souter I., et al. (2016) Urinary phthalate metabolite concentrations and reproductive outcomes among women undergoing in vitro fertilization: Results from the EARTH Study. *Environmental Health Perspectives*, 124(6): 831–839.

Hsiao P., Clavijo R.I. (2018) Adverse effects of cannabis on male reproduction. *European Urology Focus*, 4(3): 324–328.

Hu Y., Ji L., Zhang Y., et al. (2018) Organophosphate and pyrethroid pesticide exposures measured before conception and associations with time to pregnancy in Chinese couples enrolled in the Shanghai Birth Cohort. *Environmental Health Perspectives*, 126(7): 077001.

Ingaramo P.I., Guerrero Schimpf M., Milesi M.M., Luque E.H., Varayoud J. (2019) Acute uterine effects and long-term reproductive alterations in postnatally exposed female rats to a mixture of commercial formulations of endosulfan and glyphosate. *Food and Chemical Toxicology*, 134: 110832.

Kapaya M., D'Angelo D.V., Tong V.T., et al. (2019) Use of electronic vapor products before, during, and after pregnancy among women with a recent live birth—Oklahoma and Texas, 2015. *MMWR Morbidity and Mortality Weekly Report*, 68(8): 189–194.

Kasman A.M., Thoma M.E., McLain A.C., Eisenberg M.L. (2018) Association between use of marijuana and time to pregnancy in men and women: Findings from the National Survey of Family Growth. *Fertility and Sterility*, 109(5): 866–871.

Kay V.R., Chambers C., Foster W.G. (2013). Reproductive and developmental effects of phthalate diesters in females. *Critical Reviews in Toxicology*, 43(3): 200–219.

Kumar S. (2018) Occupational and environmental exposure to lead and reproductive health impairment: An overview. *Indian Journal of Occupational and Environmental Medicine*, 22(3): 128–137.

Kumar S., Sharma A. (2019). Cadmium toxicity: Effects on human reproduction and fertility. *Reviews on Environmental Health*.

Lewis R.C., Johns L.E., Meeker J.D. (2015) Serum biomarkers of exposure to perfluoralkyl substances in relation to serum testosterone and measures of thyroid function among adults and adolescents from NHANES 2011–2012. *International Journal of Environmental Research and Public Health*, 12(6): 6098–6114.

Li C., Zhao K., Zhang H., et al. (2018) Lead exposure reduces sperm quality and DNA integrity in mice. *Environmental Toxicology*, 33(5): 594–602.

Liu W., Zhou Y., Li J., et al. (2019) Parabens exposure in early pregnancy and gestational diabetes mellitus. *Environment International*, 126: 468–475.

Machtinger R., Gasking A.J., Racowsky C., et al. (2018). Urinary concentrations of biomarkers of phthalates and phthalate alternatives and IVF outcomes. *Environment International*, 111: 23–31.

Malatesta M., Boraldi F., Annova G., et al. (2008) A long-term study on female mice fed a genetically modified soybean: Effects on liver ageing. *Histochemistry and Cell Biology*, 130(5): 967–977.

Matuszczak E., Komarowska M.D., Debek W., Hermanowicz A. (2019) The impact of Bisphenol A on fertility, reproductive system, and development: A review of the literature. *International Journal of Endocrinology*, 2019: 4068717.

Messerlian C., Braun J.M., Minguez-Alarcon L., et al. (2017) Paternal and maternal urinary phthalate metabolite concentrations and birth weight of singletons conceived by subfertile couples. *Environment International*, 107: 55–64.

Minguez-Alarcon L., Gaskins A.J. (2017) Female exposure to endocrine disrupting chemicals and fecundity: A review. *Current Opinion in Obstetrics and Gynecology*, 29(4): 202–211.

Nassan F.L., Arvizu M., Minguez-Alarcon L., et al. (2019) Marijuana smoking and outcomes of infertility treatment with assisted reproductive technologies. *Human Reproduction*, 34(9): 1818–1829.

National Institute of Environmental Health Sciences. (2018) Hearing on "The Federal Role in the Toxic PFAS Crisis," Department of Health and Human Services, NIH, September 26, 2018. Retrieved from www.hsgac.senate.gov/imo/media/doc/ Birnbaum percent20Testimony.pdf December 11, 2019.

National Institute of Environmental Health Sciences (2019) Perfluoralkyl and polyfluoroalkyl substances (PFAS), National Institute of Environmental Health Science. Retrieved from www. niehs.nih.gov/health/topics/agents/pfc/index.cfm December 11, 2019.

Ozel S., Tokmak A., Aykut O., et al. (2019) Serum levels of phthalates and bisphenol-A in patients with primary ovarian insufficiency. *Gynecological Endocrinology*, 35: 364–367.

Parvez S., Gerona R.R., Proctor C., et al. (2018) Glyphosate exposure in pregnancy and shortened gestational length: A prospective Indiana birth cohort study. *Environmental Health*, 17(1): 23.

Paul R., Molto J., Ortuno N., et al. (2017) Relationship between serum dioxin-like polychlorinated biphenyls and post-testicular maturation in human sperm. *Reproductive Toxicology*, 73: 312–321.

Pednekar P.P., Gajbhiye R.K., Patil A.D., et al. (2018) Estimation of plasma levels of bisphenol-A & phthalates in fertile and infertile women by gas chromotography-mass spectrometry. *Indian Journal of Medical Research*, 148(6): 734–742.

Pizzorno J. (2018) Environmental toxins and infertility. *Integrative Medicine*, 17(2): 8–11.

Porpora M.G., Medda E., Abballe A., et al. (2009) Endometriosis and organochlorinated environmental pollutants: A case-control study on Italian women of reproductive age. *Environmental Health Perspectives*, 117(7): 1070–1075.

Rahman M.L., Zhang C., Smarr M.M., et al. (2019) Persistent organic pollutants and gestational diabetes: A multi-center prospective cohort study of healthy US women. *Environment International*, 124: 249–258.

Rashtian J., Chavkin D.E., Merhi Z. (2019) Water and soil pollution as determinant of water and food quality/contamination and its impact on female fertility. *Reproductive Biology and Endocrinology*, 17: 5.

Rattan S., Zhou C., Chiang C., Mahalingam S., Brehm E., Flaws J.A. (2017) Exposure to endocrine disruptors during adulthood: Consequences for female fertility. *Journal of Endocrinology*, 233(3): R109–R129.

Repossi A., Farabegoli F., Gazzotti T., Zironi E., Pagliuca G. (2016) Bisphenol A in edible part of seafood. *Italian Journal of Food Safety*, 5(2): 5666.

Rice K.M., Walker E.M., Wu M., Gillette C., Blough E.R. (2014). Environmental mercury and its toxic effects. *Journal of Preventative Medicine & Public Health*, 47(2): 74–83.

Rochester J.R., Bolden A.L. (2015) Bisphenol S and F: A systematic review and comparison of the hormonal activity of Bisphenol A substitutes. *Environmental Health Perspectives*, 123(7): 643–650.

Schwalfenberg G., Rodushkin I., Genuis S.J. (2018) Heavy metal contamination of prenatal vitamins. *Toxicology Reports*, 5: 390–395.

Solomon O., Yousefi P., Huen K., et al. (2017) Prenatal phthalate exposure and altered patterns of DNA methylation in cord blood. *Environmental and Molecular Mutagenesis*, 58(6): 398–410.

Thurston S.W., Mediola J., Bellamy A.R., et al. (2016) Phthalate exposure and semen quality in fertile US men. *Andrology*, 4: 632–638.

Udagawa O., Okamura K., Suzuki T., Nohara K. (2019) Arsenic Exposure and Reproductive Toxicity. In: Yamauchi H., Sun G. (Eds) *Arsenic Contamination in Asia. Current Topics in Environmental Health and Preventive Medicine.* Springer, Singapore.

United States Food and Drug Administration (2013) Phthalates. Retrieved from www.fda.gov/cosmetics/cosmetic-ingredients/phthalates December 11, 2019.

United States Department of Agriculture. (2019) Recent Trends in GE Adoption. Retrieved from www.ers.usda.gov/data-products/adoption-of-genetically-engineered-crops-in-the-us/recent-trends-in-ge-adoption.aspx November 2, 2019.

United States Environmental Protection Agency. (2019) Health Effects of Exposures to Mercury. Retrieved from www.epa.gov/mercury/health-effects-exposures-mercury November 2, 2019.

United States Environmental Protection Agency (2019). Mercury. Retrieved from www.epa.gov/mercury/advisories.htm December 11, 2019.

United States Food and Drug Administration. (2019) Consumer Q&A, Animals with Intentional Genomic Alterations. Retrieved from www.fda.gov/animal-veterinary/animals-intentional-genomic-alterations/consumer-qa November 2, 2019.

United States National Library of Medicine (2019). Phthalates. Tox Town, NIH. Retrieved from toxtown.nlm.nih.gov/chemicals-and-contaminants/phthalates December 11, 2019.

Vabre P., Gatimel N., Moreau J., et al. (2017) Environmental pollutants, a possible etiology for premature ovarian insufficiency: A narrative review of animal and human data. *Environmental Health*, 16(1): 37.

Van Bruggen A.H.C., He M.M., Shin K., et al. (2018) Environmental and health effects of the herbicide glyphosate. *The Science of the Total Environment*, 616–617: 255–268.

Wang G., DiBari J., Bind E., et al. (2019) Association between maternal exposure to lead, maternal folate status, and intergenerational risk of childhood overweight and obesity. *Journal of the American Medical Association*, 2(10): e1912343.

Wang Y.X., You L., Zeng Q., et al. (2015) Phthalate exposure and human semen quality: Results from an infertility clinic in China. *Environmental Research*, 142: 1–9.

Wetendorf M., Randall L.T., Lemma M.T., et al. (2019) E-Cigarette exposure delays implantation and causes reduced weight gain in female offspring exposed in utero. *Journal of the Endocrine Society*, 3(10): 1907–1916.

Wu H.M., Lin-Tan D.T., Wang M.L., et al. (2012) Lead level in seminal plasma may affect semen quality for men without occupational exposure to lead. *Reproductive Biology and Endocrinology*, 10: 91.

Zhang S., Tan R., Pan R., et al. (2018) Association of perfluoroalkyl and polyfluoroalkyl substances with premature ovarian insufficiency in Chinese women. *The Journal of Clinical Endocrinology and Metabolism*, 103(7): 2543–2551.

Zhou W., Zhang L., Tong C., et al. (2017) Plasma perfluoroalkyl and polyfluoroalkyl substances concentration and menstrual cycle characteristics in preconception women. *Environ Health Perspectives*, 125(6): 067012.

Acknowledgments

There are so many important people to acknowledge and thank for their role in the development of this book that it is hard to know where to begin. First, I must thank my favorite registered dieticians, Katie Bishop, RD, Kristin Criscitelli, RD, and Valerie Henderson, RD. They were instrumental to this book by assisting me doing background research, and thinking through ideas and recipes. It is a pleasure to work with such talented women. I would also like to acknowledge the ongoing support and encouragement of my literary agent, Linda Konner, who I have come to view as my literary fairy godmother. It is wonderful to work for so many years, and hopefully many more to come, with someone who I know is always constantly forward thinking, and always with my best interests at heart. This book would not have been possible without the team at Kensington. From the moment I met Denise Silvestro, my wonderful editor, I knew that this was going to be a great book. Her enthusiasm for the topic, and her vision of why this book was needed for the modern moms (and dads), made me even more excited to put this together. I would also like to thank the rest of the team, including Ann Pryor (my publicist), Shannon Plackis, Lynn Cully, Steve Zacharius, and Arthur Maisel. Lastly, I want to thank my family, who motivates me and inspires me every day. A special thank-you goes out to my daughter, Stella, who was a great help to me in testing and developing recipes. I also must thank my younger daughter, Viv, who always reminds me to take a break and play. Last but never least, a tremendous amount of gratitude goes out to my husband, Eamon, who always has been there to help me achieve my goals and gives me the confidence to do it. I pretty much couldn't do anything without you, and I like it that way. I love you.

Index

toxins, 160–76. *See also specific toxins*

trans fats, 65, 146

triggers, 48, 54–55, 56, 133

trout, 25, 34

tuna. *See* canned tuna

turkey
Easy Turmeric Turkey, Sweet Potato, and Zucchini Bowl, 73
selenium in, 41, 43
Turkey-Prosciutto Club with Homemade Chickpea Spread, 97
zinc in, 27, 42

USDA Organic label, 161

vaping, 171–72

vegans/vegetarians
omega-3 fatty acids for, 34
vitamin B_{12} for, 26
zinc for, 28

vegetables. *See also specific vegetables*
folate in, 24
happiness and, 49–50
pesticides and, 170
supplements and, 175

vegetable juices, 108
potassium in, 37, 43

Vegetarian "Meatballs" with Tomato Sauce, 79

vitamins. *See also specific vitamins*
supplements, 175–76

vitamin A, 38–39, 43
recommended daily intake, 38, 43
sources of, 38, 43

vitamin B_6, 28–29, 42
recommended daily intake, 28, 42
sources of, 28, 42, 95

vitamin B9. *See* folate/folic acid

vitamin B_{12}, 25–27, 42
recommended daily intake, 25, 42
sources of, 25, 26, 42

vitamin C, 39–40, 43
iron absorption and, 32
nonheme iron absorption, 31, 32
recommended daily intake, 39, 43
sources of, 39, 43, 74, 75, 83, 91, 108

vitamin D, 36–37, 43
recommended daily intake, 36, 43
sources of, 36–37, 43

vitamin D supplements, 37, 176

vitamin E, sources of, 94

vitamin K, sources of, 67, 83, 91

Waffles with Honey-Sweetened Frozen Yogurt, 155

weight, 8, 14–16
self-medicating with food, 50–51

weight gain. *See also* obesity
dopamine reward system and, 53
processed foods and, 53, 58

weight loss
fertility and, 15–16
keto diet for, 17–18

wheat bran, 61–64
Banana-Bran Pancakes, 63–64
magnesium in, 29, 42, 61